T0369232

It Was a Privilege to Care for Her

BY

KEITH A. KLAFEHN

Order this book online at www.trafford.com
or email orders@trafford.com

Most Trafford titles are also available at major online book retailers.

© Copyright 2009 KEITH A. KLAFEHN.
All rights reserved. No part of this publication may be reproduced, stored in a retrieval
system, or transmitted, in any form or by any means, electronic, mechanical, photocopying,
recording, or otherwise, without the written prior permission of the author.

Print information available on the last page.

ISBN: 978-1-4251-8997-6 (sc)

Because of the dynamic nature of the Internet, any web addresses or links contained in
this book may have changed since publication and may no longer be valid. The views
expressed in this work are solely those of the author and do not necessarily reflect the views
of the publisher, and the publisher hereby disclaims any responsibility for them.

Any people depicted in stock imagery provided by Thinkstock are models,
and such images are being used for illustrative purposes only.
Certain stock imagery © Thinkstock.

Trafford rev. 06/23/2015

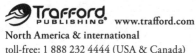 www.trafford.com

North America & international
toll-free: 1 888 232 4444 (USA & Canada)
fax: 812 355 4082

THIS BOOK IS DEDICATED TO

Mark and Kay
Children of Muriel and Keith

Kaitlyn, Kenton, Meagan, and Emma
Oma's and Grandpa's Grandchildren

TABLE OF CONTENTS

I will weep when you are weeping
When you laugh I'll laugh with you.
I will share your joy and sorrow
'Til we've seen this journey through.*

*"The Servant Song," Richard Gillard, © 1977 Scripture in Song/ Maranatha! Music/ASCAP. All rights administered by Music Services, Inc.) All rights reserved. Used by permission.

INTRODUCTION

There are over one million new cases of cancer diagnosed in the United States on an annual basis and the number seems to be on the increase. In contrast, great strides are being made in this country in the effort to eliminate cancer. The American Cancer Society and Susan G. Komen for the Cure are but two of the organizations that provide research funds in an ongoing search to cure cancer. Many victims of cancer have been helped by this research and have become survivors. But not all of those persons who get breast cancer survive the disease.

The subject of this book, Muriel E. J. Klafehn, is one of those persons. With the exception of the patient's loved ones, those individuals who administer to cancer patients, the oncologists and their staffs, hospice personnel, and visiting nurses who tend these individuals, most people do not realize what those cancer patients go through as they try to prolong their lives.

This book has been written to provide a picture of the path that one individual has taken, from diagnosis to death. How is the knowledge that one has breast cancer handled by the individual as well as those around her? How does the loss of a breast affect one's life? How does one handle the first metastasis? The second? How does one handle a three to six month prognosis? How is one affected when going from 20 mg of OxyContin three times a day to 300 mg three times a day?

During an interview regarding his wife's cancer, Rick Warren, the author of *The Purpose Driven Life*, tells us you can focus on your purposes or you can focus on your problems, and he suggests that focusing on your problems is self-centered. Muriel Klafehn chose to focus on her purpose, exclaiming not *Why me?* but *Why not me?* She judged that God had a purpose in permitting her to have cancer and to even lose her life as a result of the disease. I have tried to convey her message of purpose throughout the book and it is to be hoped that as you read, you will have a sense of Muriel's resolve to be God's instrument to strengthen the faith of others. In the process of dying there are many "lasts." The last birthday. The last anniversary. The last Thanksgiving. The last Christmas. The last time you drive the car. The last time you see your sister. The last time you see your children and grandchildren. When friends come to visit is it the last time you will see them? Maybe dying should be private and reserved only for family and friends. However, because dying happens to everybody, I believe that those individuals who have been diagnosed with cancer and those who care for them should be aware of one woman's "adventure."

< 1 >
THE "ADVENTURE" BEGINS

Thursday, September 24, 1998

Muriel was just fifteen minutes late but it felt like an hour. My 11:00 meeting with my Stephen Ministry care receiver had been canceled, so I waited at home for her to return from her doctor's appointment. It wasn't a routine visit and so time moved in slow motion as my mind overworked itself.

Muriel's appointment this morning was with her oncological gynecologist, Dr. John Karlen. She had seen him earlier in the week to have him look at her right breast. She had been having some soreness and wanted to get it checked out. Dr. Karlen had taken one look at her breast and ushered her down the hall to Dr. Flynn's office where he completed a needle biopsy. The results would be available today.

She was expected home by 11:30. When the telephone finally rang at nearly quarter to 12, I snatched it off its hook before the first ring had ended. "Hello?"

"Hello sweetie," Muriel said, "I thought you would be at church."

"Well, my eleven o'clock canceled and I've been waiting here to find out about your biopsy. Are you still at the office? What happened?"

"I'd rather talk to you in person. I'm at the church. Come over and I'll fill you in."

"That doesn't sound good to me," I added nervously.

"No, everything is fine. You're going to play bridge anyway so just come to the church and we can talk then."

I pressed her a bit but soon relented when she insisted that I come to the church.

"I guess I don't have a choice in the matter. I'll see you in a few minutes."

I said goodbye quietly and left immediately for the church. Given Muriel's reluctance to tell me anything my thoughts were for the worst. As I walked to the garage I had a mental image of a neon sign flashing "CANCER" in big red letters. With my heart beating a little faster, I backed the car out of the garage and began the drive to our church.

There are nine traffic lights between our house and the church. The first one I encountered was green and I said a prayer of thanks as I continued my drive. However, the next two lights were red. I sat patiently willing them to change so that I could continue on. When they turned green, I tried to maintain the proper speed to time the lights and avoid any further delay as my anxiety mounted. My efforts were to no avail though as I waited through four more red lights sandwiched around two greens. By the time I finally arrived at church, I practically sprinted from the car in search of Muriel.

I found her in the church office speaking with Rita Cargill, the church secretary. She bid Rita farewell as she calmly took hold of my hand and said, "Let's go out to the meditation area where we can be alone." We walked quietly hand in hand and seated ourselves on a bench facing each other.

Muriel could tell from the pleading look on my face that I needed to know what had transpired in Dr. Karlen's office. She said, "Sweetie, everything is not all right. The biopsy indicated the presence of breast cancer and I'll be going to the hospital in the morning where Dr. Flynn will remove my right breast."

Tears instantly welled up in my eyes and spilled down my cheeks. It felt as if someone had punched me in the gut and knocked the wind out of me. Muriel held me close and said, "We'll be all right but I want you to promise me two things. One, that you will go and play bridge this afternoon and two, that you will take me to El Campesino for dinner tonight."

I halfheartedly agreed and, sensing my hesitation, she added, "When Dr. Karlen told me I had cancer, I wasn't surprised. I had expected it." My expression in response to this revelation more than made up for her lack of surprise. This was a piece of information she had not shared with me.

Muriel added, "I'm not angry with God. I am not even asking *Why me?* When Dr. Karlen told me I had cancer I prayed to God, not to heal me, but to give me His peace, and as soon as I had prayed, God gave me peace. I'm completely at ease with what has happened and from here on out this will be considered my 'adventure.'"

I was pained, overwhelmed by the idea that I could possibly lose her. Almost as quickly as these thoughts had overcome me, I could see Muriel's faith shining through and I took solace in her reaction.

"I do not want to hear anyone talking about 'battling cancer,'" she continued. "I hate that term because a battle implies that there's a winner and a loser, and as far as I am concerned if I become cancer-free I will be able to stay here on Earth and spend more time with you. And if I die, I will go home to be with the Lord. It's a win-win situation."

We rose from the bench and I gave Muriel a long hug and a kiss. I walked her to her car and she left for home while I remained behind to play bridge as promised. She was going to call her sister Judith and our two children Mark and Kay to let them know that she has cancer and will be having surgery in the morning. Our children and her sister reside in the Dallas area of Texas so there is little chance anyone other than myself will be able to accompany her to surgery in the morning. Muriel is quite comfortable with the fact that I will be the only one present.

I stopped in the office briefly to share the news with Rita, but apparently Muriel had already informed her so she gave me a hug and said both of us would be in her prayers. My next stop was the fellowship hall where I informed all of my fellow games players about Muriel's breast cancer and pending operation, and that she had made me promise to stay and play bridge. So I told them, "Here I am." We began to play and I received many words of comfort and promises of prayer support.

Muriel knew that playing bridge was one of my passions, and until I retired I had not often played. I had learned to play when I was in the military back in 1955. I played some in college, but Muriel didn't play and I was reluctant to go out in the evening, alone, just to play bridge. Fellowship, Fun, and Games met every other Thursday and then we who were bridge players decided to meet on the off Thursday as well. Since joining, I had been enjoying bridge every week. One of my

Thursday cohorts also invited me to play in a friendly game on Monday mornings at the community center in Cuyahoga Falls, Ohio. Since I was generally out to a men's Bible class that morning, I just continued on gratefully to play bridge on Mondays with Muriel's blessing.

In the evening I honored the second half of my earlier promise and Muriel and I went out to dinner at El Campesino, a favorite Mexican restaurant in Stow, where we each had a margarita and enjoyed their chicken chimichangas. We discussed the events of the day and the "adventure" on which we were embarking.

Later that evening we nestled close together in her waterbed finding great comfort in our togetherness. As Muriel drifted off to sleep, I returned to my bed and settled down to a fitful rest. Since we are empty nesters we had two extra bedrooms and prior to Muriel's retirement we had agreed to sleep apart. The waterbed was much too warm to suit me and Muriel generally read in the evening which made it difficult for me to fall asleep until the light was out. I was a chronic snorer so sleeping apart provided uninterrupted quiet time for Muriel to get her rest. Also, if I chose to stay up late, my coming to bed would not disturb her. I think we both ultimately slept better and there was always a standing invitation to share time in each other's bed enjoying connubial bliss.

Since Muriel was having surgery, it was a requirement of her insurance company to have a second opinion. Dr. Flynn had agreed to contact Mutual Health Services Company to take care of that. Before leaving the hospital on Thursday, Muriel had pre-registered and gone through all of the pre-admission testing. That would enable her to arrive in the morning and go directly to surgery.

Friday, September 25, 1998

We were up early and since Muriel was due to have an operation she was not allowed to have anything to eat or drink. As a show of solidarity, I wished to skip breakfast as well, but Muriel insisted that I eat something. I thus had my usual bowl of cereal and cup of coffee and glanced briefly at the paper. Muriel had packed a bag the night before and was ready to depart by 6:00. I gathered up some reading material and we drove the eight miles to the hospital where she was scheduled for a 7:15 surgery with Dr. Flynn. We had little conversation on the way in but one thing in particular she said helped to lift both our spirits. "God's peace is still with me and I'm ready to have this breast removed and get on with my life."

4

I took Muriel to pre-op and waited while she changed into the proverbial back-opening hospital gown. All of her belongings were placed into a plastic bag and put in my care. The last item she gave up was her glasses and she was not very happy about that as her ability to see without them is almost non-existent. I kissed her goodbye and headed to the surgery waiting room.

I reported to the reception desk in the waiting area and the receptionist matched my name to Muriel's on her list. I let her know where I would be in the room should I need to be contacted. I found a seat and took out the current issue of *Sports Illustrated* and began to read.

Needless to say, it was difficult to concentrate on what I was reading and I got up to get a cup of coffee. All of this waiting stuff was brand new to me. With the exception of giving birth to our two children, this was the first time that Muriel had ever been hospitalized. I sipped my coffee and continued to attempt to read. Periodically a doctor would appear in the waiting area and a family would be called out to meet with the doctor to be apprised of the status of their loved one. Sometimes these conferences were held behind closed doors, and one can only assume the news the doctor would convey was not good.

At 8:30 Pastor Johnson, from our church, arrived to lend me moral support and to offer up prayers for Muriel's safe surgery. He soon departed and I was once again left to myself to contemplate Muriel's surgery and to read as best I could. I took a quick trip to the men's room to dispose of the cup of coffee I had drunk, then back to my seat to wait.

Dr. Flynn appeared at 9:15 and I was summoned to meet with him. Thankfully Muriel's surgery had been successful. In a clinical manner he relayed what had happened. "We performed a radical mastectomy and the ten lymph nodes on the right side were removed. The lymph nodes and breast will be sent to the pathology laboratory for further analysis." In parting he said, "She's resting in the recovery room. You're welcome to go in and sit with her."

When I walked into the room, Muriel was still under the influence of her anesthesia. She looked so peaceful lying there and I reached out and held her hand and kissed her on the cheek. About a half hour after I had arrived Muriel came out of her groggy state and was happy to see me and to get her glasses back. I joked with her to break the ice. "Are you happier to see me or your glasses?"

"Well without my glasses I can't see you, so I suppose the glasses," she quipped, smiling a bit yet wincing.

5

I tried to smile back but my look of concern superseded that. "How are you feeling?"

"Considering what just happened, I actually feel reasonably good. Sore, but not too bad."

This time I managed a smile and put my hand over hers. I silently offered a prayer of thanks for her having come through the surgery all right and a second prayer for a speedy recovery. The nurse came around and checked her vital signs and let us know she was ready to be moved to her hospital room.

In 20 minutes, with the help of a volunteer, she was moved to her room in the oncology section of the hospital. It was a typical hospital room, two beds with the mobile tray holders, two chairs, two televisions, and the wraparound curtains. There was a closet where I deposited her bag of clothing. There was also a bathroom for patient or visitor use. Muriel closed her eyes and appeared to be ready to doze off. "Get some rest," I suggested. "I'll be back this evening." She smiled again as I kissed her goodbye. With mixed feelings I departed to take care of phone calls and other tasks around home.

The first thing I did when I arrived home was to call both of our children and Muriel's sister in Texas to let them know that the surgery was successful and she was recovering. I also called my two sisters, one in Florida and one in Colorado, and let them know about Muriel's "adventure." I then took time to shower and eat dinner before heading back to the hospital to see Muriel.

She was attempting to eat her dinner when I came in and I crossed the room to give her a kiss. I could see she was unhappy. "Look what they fed me. Soup, a fruit drink, and Jell-O. Yuck!" The meal did look unappealing but she tried her best to finish it all. I think I had been there all of four minutes when all that she had eaten decided to reappear. I tried to get the basin up to her mouth but some ended up down the front of her and onto the sheets and blanket. She pressed her button to summon her nurse. I emptied the basin while the nurse outfitted Muriel with a new gown and with the help of another nurse, stripped and remade the bed.

I think that some of the peace that Muriel had prayed for enveloped me, because in the past if someone in the family had thrown up I would have thrown up with them or at least would have left the room retching. Instead I had reached for the basin and actually held it while Muriel vomited, and then I even emptied the basin.

It was the first time since the adventure began that I too had felt the peace for which Muriel had prayed. Muriel was impressed knowing how I had always been in the past. "Thank you honey. I know how hard that must have been for you." She smiled at me.

"Not nearly as hard as what you are handling," I answered, looking deeply into her eyes. "It is amazing what God can do in your life if you just let Him." I smiled back and hugged her tightly.

We quietly watched a little television but as the evening wore on, Muriel began to tire so I prepared to depart. Muriel had been cleared to leave the following morning.

"I'll call you to let you know when to come pick me up," she said.

"I'll be waiting to hear from you." I gave her another hug and kiss. I could clearly see the effect of the Vicodin she had been given earlier as she was dropping off to sleep when I walked out the door.

I arrived home to an empty house, watched some television, and climbed in bed to read. My prayers for the evening included great thankfulness for the successful surgery, for the peace that enveloped Muriel and that I too had felt, and for the first steps in restoring order into our lives once again.

Saturday, September 26, 1998

I woke up early to an unusually empty home, making me all the more eager to bring Muriel home. I exercised, ate breakfast, and read the newspaper while I waited for her call. At 9:30 the phone rang. It was Muriel offering a warm greeting. "Good morning sweetheart. You can pick me up around 11:00."

"I'm looking forward to it," I said. We spoke for a few minutes and I ended the call with, "See you soon. I love you." I straightened up the kitchen and departed for the hospital at 10:15. I detoured to the pharmacy to pick up the prescription for Vicodin, which I had dropped off on my way home the previous night. I parked the car in the parking deck and made my way to Muriel's room.

She was dressed and ready to go but had not gotten her going-home instructions. I greeted her with a hug and a kiss and asked if she had gotten a good night's sleep. She answered, "I did but I'm ready to go home."

"And I'm more than ready to have you home. It was lonely without you this morning," I confessed.

Luckily, within minutes of my arrival, the nurse came into the room and provided going-home instructions: Vicodin every four hours as needed for pain; empty drain as needed; strip tubing three times a day; and record all drainage.

She also told Muriel that she could resume taking her other medications and added, "Dr. Flynn's resident suggested you call on Monday to make an appointment with Dr. Flynn for Tuesday to have your dressing changed." The nurse also gave her the name of a support group, Reach for Recovery. Muriel was put into a wheelchair and I headed for the parking deck to bring the car around to the pick-up point. Since she was ambulatory she moved easily from the wheelchair to the car. I got her home and settled her into her La-Z-Boy and suggested that she rest for a while.

We were scheduled that evening for the first concert of the subscription season by the Akron Symphony Orchestra, and we had also made plans to go out for dinner before the concert. I felt uneasy about planning such a busy evening so soon and asked, "Do you think it's a good idea to go out tonight?"

Muriel replied, "Of course it's a good idea. I just want everything to get back to normal and eating out and going to the concert is part of normal."

I made her a grilled cheese sandwich for lunch and she dozed until it was time to get ready to go out. She managed to shower without mishap and I participated in the stripping of the tubing, recording the number of cc of liquid that was removed. She was ready to go at 5:15.

We left for dinner and ate at Michael Treacaso's Italian Restaurant, a place close to the site of the concert, E. J. Thomas Hall, so we wouldn't be rushed after dinner. We were seated in a booth beside the cash register and enjoyed the Italian cuisine. We each had a glass of wine with our meal which may not have been the best idea. I got up to pay the bill and as I was signing the credit card voucher, out of the corner of my eye I could see Muriel stand. I then heard a "thunk" and turned to see Muriel in a crumpled heap on the floor. The sound had been of her head hitting the edge of the table as she fainted.

I rushed to her side as did the owner. We got her back into the booth we had occupied and a waitress got a cold compress which I put on her forehead. She was revived almost immediately and was embarrassed at what had happened. The knock on the table had opened a small cut on the back of her head, so I took her to the ladies room and cleaned up the blood that was matted in her hair. After about five minutes we were ready to leave. The owner, a former student of mine, was very concerned for her well-being. "I know she's tough, but please call me if anything happens."

As we began our walk to E. J. Thomas Hall I said, "We should forfeit our tickets and head home." She forcefully replied, "Absolutely not!" So we began our slow walk to the concert hall. The enjoyment of symphonic music had always been a part of our relationship. Muriel was introduced to classical music as a youngster when her father would take her to hear the New York Philharmonic. During the summers of her youth, the Philadelphia Orchestra under the direction of Eugene Ormandy would come to Englewood, New Jersey where she would go to hear that great orchestra.

My first exposure to classical music came when I was in the military and heard the 7th Army Symphony Orchestra at a concert given in Bamberg, Germany. They played two pieces, *Scheherazade* by Rimsky-Korsakov and The Suite from *Lt. Keje* by Prokofiev. To this day those two pieces are still among my all-time favorite classical pieces.

When we moved to Ohio in 1969, it seemed only proper to have season tickets for the great Cleveland Orchestra as well as our own Akron Symphony. We were very fortunate to be in attendance at E. J. Thomas Hall when the Royal Concertgeboew Orchestra of Amsterdam was on a tour and we heard the Second Symphony of Rachmaninoff. Muriel would always count the time that we spent listening to that renowned piece as a defining moment in our relationship. We had been privileged to hear that piece several times since, and each time we were transfixed as we listened to the nuances of the piece and the individual sonorities.

The conductor this evening was Eric Benjamin, the assistant conductor of the Akron Symphony Orchestra, and the whole concert had an Irish and Scottish theme. The program began with *Four Scottish Dances* by Malcolm Arnold, followed by "Irish Tune from County Derry" (Danny Boy) sung by tenor Pat Flynn. Two more pieces followed before intermission, "Marches and Airs" arranged by Benjamin, and *An Orkney Wedding, with Sunrise* by Peter Maxwell Davies. For the latter piece, Bruce Gbur took center stage in his Scottish kilt and played his bagpipe. After intermission we heard the *The Hebrides* Overture by Mendelssohn and concluded the evening with Stanford's Symphony No. 3 in F Minor, Op. 28 (*Irish*) 2nd and 4th movts. We greatly enjoyed the music, but I think Muriel was happy to get home and into her waterbed. It had been quite a day.

Sunday, September 27, 1998

"Good morning sweetheart," Muriel cheerily greeted me. She joined me at the kitchen table and began to drink the cup of coffee I had made for her. I returned the greeting and asked her how she felt. "I feel great, but I'm a little sore where the breast was removed." The sleep must have been good for her because she did look pretty chipper.

"Do you think you can direct the Chorale this morning?" I asked.

"Absolutely, I wouldn't miss it for anything."

Muriel is the director of the Chorale at our church, Redeemer Lutheran in Cuyahoga Falls, and we were scheduled to sing at the first service. We dressed for church and were soon on our way. Of course many members of the Chorale knew she had been in the hospital on Friday and were amazed that she would even attempt to come to church and, no less, contemplate directing. She was bombarded with comments like "Are your sure you should be doing this?" "Sue can get us through the piece." "Kathy can start us and stop us." "Why don't you just sit this one out?"

But direct she did and I think in doing so bolstered the faith of many members of the Chorale. The pastor said public prayers of thanksgiving for Muriel's successful surgery and continued blessings on her full recovery. For many members of the congregation it was the first they knew of her operation. We went to Communion together and returned hand in hand up the center aisle to smiles and nods of many members of the congregation.

The text for Pastor Johnson's sermon was Isaiah 40:31, *"But those who hope in the Lord will renew their strength. They will soar on wings like eagles; they will run and not grow weary, they will walk and not be faint."* As the sermon unfolded, it was pointed out that in the time of a storm eagles will rise above the storm and just soar on the thermals until the storm has diminished. We discussed that aspect on our way home from church.

"God has already delivered me a lifeline and now He has given me a mantra," she said.

"How do you mean?" I asked curiously.

"He granted me peace for my adventure," she answered, "and now I'm going to soar above the storm."

Monday, September 28, 1998

It had been a general practice that since Muriel's retirement I would try to accompany her on all of her medical appointments. However, this goal was not always met because of my own commitments.

Today I incorporated the additional task into my routine of making the appropriate appointments as well. So I called Dr. Flynn's office to make an appointment for Muriel for Thursday, the first of October.

Tuesday, September 29, 1998

I called Regina Brett to see if she might be willing to have a joint column with the husband of a breast cancer patient. She was a columnist for our local newspaper, the *Akron Beacon Journal*, and had done a wonderful series of articles on what had happened in her life when she had breast cancer. She seemed receptive to the idea but she also left me with the impression that she would probably not call me back.

Thursday, October 1, 1998

We began our day by attending a meeting of our Stephen Ministry leaders that was scheduled for 9:30. I had an appointment with my care receiver at 11:00, and after lunch I accompanied Muriel to her 1:30 appointment with Dr. Flynn. We had previously arranged to spend a week at Virginia Beach in North Carolina, so we had begun our preparations for our departure and were seeking approval for our scheduled travel. The doctor checked her incision, removed the drainage tubing, and then replaced the wrapping. In parting he said, "Have a relaxing vacation. Your time away should help the healing process." This was great to hear as I think it was important to both Muriel and me that he sent us off with his blessing. We also got a prescription for hydrocodone, the generic form of Vicodin, should Muriel experience any pain while we were away.

Before we departed we spent some time with the receptionist as we sought out an oncologist to treat Muriel. We were provided with three names and decided to make an appointment with Dr. Joseph Koenig. I called his office when we got home and the earliest we could see him was October 21. The prospect of having to wait nearly three weeks to see the doctor did not set well with me, but Muriel just made the judgment, "This is the way it's supposed to be so let's just wait until then to see him."

Friday, October 2, 1998

In preparation for our week in North Carolina we went grocery shopping. I took care of stopping the mail, arranging for our papers to be accumulated, and notifying the police that we would be out of town for one week. For the most part the day was spent preparing for our trip. In the evening we went out to dinner and then attended a Cleveland Orchestra concert at Severance Hall. Christoph von Dohnányi, the musical director of the orchestra, selected two pieces by Ives, *Central Park in the Dark* and the world premiere of Emerson Concerto, with Alan Feinberg the pianist. After intermission we thoroughly enjoyed a performance of Beethoven's Symphony No. 3 (*Eroica*).

Because we arrive home so late from these concerts, nearly 11:30 each time, we had made the decision that this would be the last year for season tickets for the Cleveland Orchestra. They may be touted as "the best band in the land" and we have been supporters and concertgoers for many years, but we decided to put our support dollars toward the Akron Symphony Orchestra and continue to enjoy the concerts a little closer to home.

Saturday, October 3, 1998

It has been one week since Muriel came home from the hospital. She continues to exhibit great resilience, so today we attended the wedding and reception of Brenda Blanchard, the daughter of Barb Blanchard, one of the members of our Chorale. The service was beautiful and it allowed us to silently renew our vows and the closeness we were experiencing as we continued on Muriel's adventure. We also enjoyed the reception and even danced when the music was from our era. We had courted to Johnny Mathis and "The Twelfth of Never" and later, Kenny Rogers singing "Through the Years" and Henry Mancini's "Softly, as I Leave You." Perhaps it shows our age, but all of the acoustic guitars and keyboards were not our cup of tea. However, when a slow piece was played we took advantage of it.

Sunday, October 11, 1998

We left last Sunday for a week at Virginia Beach. The accommodations were more than adequate. I was in charge of the cooking although it was not a difficult task as we had prepared a menu prior to our departure and had purchased all of the ingredients in anticipation of our trip. All we had to do was pick up milk, salad, and some goodies.

It was a wonderful week, just what the doctor ordered I suppose. I played golf a couple of times with Muriel's blessing. I was concerned about leaving her for the four hours it would take me to play. However, she had brought several books and was very content to relax and read and rest. We walked on the beach each day, and she seemed to grow stronger with each passing day. I picked up white polished stones on our daily beach walks with the intent of having several of them put on a chain or strung as a necklace for Muriel. When we got home from Virginia Beach, we put all of the stones in a small wicker basket and placed them on our coffee table in the family room where they would serve as a reminder of our time together at Virginia Beach. I sorted out eight of the smaller stones and took them to a jeweler to see if he could string them up for me, but unfortunately he was unable to do that.

Time spent at the beach was a panacea to Muriel, very therapeutic. Muriel had been going to the beach with her parents since she was a youngster and absolutely loved it. Several years ago we had purchased a time-share week in Myrtle Beach and returned each year for a time of rejuvenation. She had often told me that if she should die before me she wanted to be cremated and then have her ashes strewn at the ocean. She had agreed to spread mine at the golf course.

Monday, October 12, 1998

One of the things Muriel had done while we were in North Carolina was to prepare her menus for the month, and the air of normalcy continued. You need to understand that Muriel is extremely well organized. As she often told me, she had to be, to juggle her teaching schedule, correcting papers, and her responsibilities at home and church. She absolutely detested coming home from teaching and then deciding what she was to have for dinner.

So each month she prepared dinner menus for each day of every week and would then make her shopping list according to the items she needed to make those meals, completing it by adding the staples we needed around the house. The meal lineup included chicken, fish, and turkey, with a mix of meat and vegetarian meals to complete the month. This list was then typed up and posted on the refrigerator so I could see at a glance what we were to have for dinner each day of the month.

Compiling the shopping list was not the end of the process. She would then put all the items in order so we could enter the store and go up one aisle, down the next, up the next and so on, then move on to the cash register and out the door. She also noted on her shopping list if she had any coupons that could be used. Muriel always clipped coupons and filed them in a file box by category. Thus the box was always consulted when making out the shopping list. Initially the coupons with expired dates were eliminated and then those that could be used on this shopping trip were paper clipped together and clipped to her shopping list. We rarely got any items that were not on her list. She also maintained an additional list of fresh items to be purchased each Sunday when we came home from church.

So today, with her shopping list and coupons in hand, we went shopping at the Finast grocery store and, as usual, it was into the store, up one aisle, down the next, up the next, etc., to the check out, and out the door. No extras, just what was on the list. It was a sight to see and she hadn't lost a step. When we got home, all of the items were put into their proper place on the shelves in the basement. Her inventory system was outstanding and would have put many businesses to shame. We never ran out of anything, it seemed, because as the last item was brought up from the basement it would be placed on the "to get" list for the next shopping trip.

After lunch Muriel had a 1:30 appointment with Dr. Waugh, her regular internist. His office was in Kent right on Water Street. We parked in the back and went down the steps leading into the National City Bank building. Dr. Waugh's office was on the second floor. There were several chairs in the 10- by 15-foot reception room. There was a glass window on the far wall where each patient reported when he or she came in. After checking in we both took a seat and waited to be called into the examination room.

We had probably been there only five minutes when Dottie, Dr. Waugh's nurse, called Muriel in to be examined. I accompanied her into the office and observed as Dottie took her blood pressure and pulse and then seated us in the examination room. When Dr. Waugh came in, Muriel brought him up to date on all of the health-related events that had transpired in her life since she had last visited him. The doctor did the usual examination of her throat, nose, and ears, listened to her heart and lungs, then provided her with new prescriptions for her Maxzide and Lescol. We departed with a new appointment scheduled in two months.

Friday, October 16, 1998

"Hurray, we did it," I cheered.

"Did you expect differently?" Muriel asked, grinning.

"No, I guess not," I answered reflectively.

"Soaring above the storm, right? Faith brings you to high places, like this," she said.

"True, and here's to many more," I said as I closed the gap between us and offered her a kiss. "We'll get our medallions yet," I added. I turned to enjoy the view with her for a quiet moment. We had just finished hiking Highbridge Trail in Cuyahoga Falls. For the past dozen years we had been involved in the Fall Hiking Spree held at the Akron Metro Parks. If you hiked eight of the thirteen assigned trails you would receive a medallion which was added to the hiking staff that you received the first time you hiked. Each year we chose to do all thirteen

14

trails, and since Muriel was feeling in good shape this morning, she wanted to add to our tally to make sure we still got all of our trails in.

The trails are graded by difficulty, i.e., one, two, and three, with three being the most difficult. Difficulty was emphasized by the amount of elevation one had to traverse in the process of completing the trail. Highbridge Trail is in Cascade Valley Metro Park and is rated a two. It was number seven of thirteen and it felt great to get over the halfway mark. I suspect we were a little slower than in past trail hikes, but we had completed it in good form. Seven down, six to go.

Saturday, October 17, 1998

Another busy day. Muriel and I were both Stephen Ministers and had also been trained as Stephen Leaders. Today we were part of a Stephen Ministry workshop at our church. Many pastors and laypersons in our area had been invited to come to find out what Stephen Ministry was all about. We were both involved in leading sessions and making presentations. The workshop included a buffet lunch prepared by Pastor Johnson's wife and her committee.

We relaxed briefly in the late afternoon and then went to an Akron Symphony Orchestra concert. The conductor for the evening was Louis Lane, director emeritus of the Orchestra. The program began with *Variations on a Theme by Haydn*, Op. 56 by Johannes Brahms, followed by Kodály's *Háry János* Suite with Alex Udvary on cello. After intermission Louis Lortie was the pianist for the Piano Concerto No. 1 in E-flat Major by Liszt. The final piece by the orchestra was the rousing *Capriccio Espagnol*, Op. 34 by Rimsky-Korsakov. Climbing into the waterbed that night was a welcome relief as we briefly shared our togetherness.

Sunday, October 18, 1998

We went to church as usual and stopped at Acme to pick up the fresh items on Muriel's shopping list. After lunch we decided to earn our medallions by hiking trail number eight at Firestone Metro Park. It was rated a one so Muriel did quite well. I silently wondered if this would be the first year that we would be unable to complete all thirteen trails by the end of November, or for that matter, if we would go far beyond the minimum number of trails to get our medallions. I judged that with some twos and threes yet to do and chemotherapy on the horizon it would certainly be quite difficult to accomplish.

Monday, October 19, 1998

Today we got a call from our son Mark to inform us that grandchild number four had arrived, weighing in at 6 pounds, 4 ounces and measuring 21 inches long. Both the mother, Cathy, and child, Emma Catherine, were doing well. I think Muriel was particularly pleased at the name since her mother's name was Emma, but she really liked the combination of Emma Catherine.

Tuesday, October 20, 1998

Muriel and I ate lunch at Applebee's, one of our favorite restaurants, prior to her 1:30 appointment with Dr. Flynn. He checked out her incision for the last time. He had also received the pathology report and indicated that all ten of the lymph nodes had been cancerous. He also informed us that Muriel had a Grade III tumor. "There are four grades of which four is worst, but Grade III is certainly not a death sentence. We are just grading the type of cancer and its growth rate."

On our drive home we spent time speculating on the meaning of the pathology report. The next day we were to meet with Dr. Koenig and we judged he would have a more definitive prognosis.

< 2 >
CHEMOTHERAPY: ROUND ONE

Wednesday, October 21, 1998

Today Muriel is to meet with her oncologist Dr. Joseph Koenig at 10:00. Dr. Koenig, together with Drs. Trochelman and Ross, comprise the group known collectively as Summit Oncology Associates, Inc. They are located in Akron on the second floor of 92 Arch Street, a physician's office building, attached to Summa Health System.

We arrived at 9:30 because it was necessary for us to complete some paperwork prior to seeing the doctor. The entry door to the waiting area was on the right corner of the room, which appeared to be about 25 feet long and 15 feet wide. There was a building pillar about two-thirds of the way down the room which made the room seem congested. There was a door on the right-hand wall which led to the examination area, and the wall facing you as you entered the room had two large sliding glass windows about ten feet apart. One was the admission window and the other was the payment and appointment window.

Chairs and love seats accented by tables and lamps were dispersed around the room, giving it a comfortable feel I hadn't felt initially. The tables held magazines for reading while waiting to see the doctor. Recessed overhead fluorescent lighting completed the warmth of the room.

Walking into the office was not a shock but was somewhat over-whelming. There were few vacant seats and the individuals experiencing chemotherapy were evident. The women suffering from hair loss were arrayed in turbans, and other sorts of head-covering apparel. The men with prominent bald heads were more obvious. Muriel took a seat by me. While she completed her paperwork, I sat there astonished by the damage that cancer was wreaking on other humans in this room. Was Muriel to be a part of this scene? Was she going to lose her hair? My thoughts snapped back to the present when Muriel arose to turn in her paperwork. We took out our reading material and bided our time. It was 10:10 when we heard Muriel's name being called.

We followed the nurse who had summoned Muriel through the door and entered a room similar in size to the reception area but turned 90 degrees. Immediately to the right was a small room which served as an overflow room for those patients having chemotherapy. Next to it was a door that entered into the hematology area. The facing wall contained a long counter with cabinets above and fluorescent lighting under the cabinets. There were three telephones spaced out on the counter and two of them were being used by nurses, carrying on the business, one assumes, of speaking with patients. On the immediate left as you entered the room was another glass window with a technician, seated behind the window, who helped arrange for various scans as prescribed by the doctors. By the glass window was a scale and then a doorway to the records office. Then came a hallway that went in both directions and was separated from the counter area by a divider that was open at the top. To the right, down the hallway, were physician's examination rooms and, way at the end, accounting offices and other rooms associated with the practice. Down the hallway to the left was an archival room. The left side of the room we were in had a door that led to the chemotherapy room.

Inside the door to the reception area we were met by Laura, one of Dr. Koenig's nursing staff. Muriel was weighed (120 pounds) and measured (5' 2"), and then taken to an examination room. It was a typical examination room, approximately 10 feet by 15 feet, with a sink, two chairs, cabinets, an examination table with a step stool, and a cushioned physician's stool with rollers.

Muriel provided Laura with a typewritten list of all of her doctors, as well as a complete listing of all the medications she was taking at the time—further evidence of Muriel's preparedness and organization. Laura added the sheets to Muriel's file and then took her blood pressure (122/78) and pulse (72). Lastly she handed Muriel a paper blouse and asked her to remove the clothing on her upper body and put on the blouse. She indicated that Dr. Koenig would be in shortly.

Muriel removed her clothes, slipped into the paper blouse and took a seat on the examination table. Dr. Koenig arrived shortly after that and introduced himself as he walked to the sink to wash his hands. He was tall, around 6' 2", and slight of build. He had on a shirt and tie and the typical white lab coat. After discussing Muriel's medical history Dr. Koenig offered his broad recommendation. "Given that the pathology report indicated that all ten lymph nodes were cancerous, I want to take a very aggressive approach to the treatment of your cancer." At the time we simply nodded, unaware of just what such an approach might entail. I was naturally apprehensive but did my best not to show it. If Muriel shared my apprehension, she too suppressed it as her expression was one of calmness.

Dr. Koenig had Muriel lie down on the examination table and he then performed an examination of the breast area. When he finished he said, "We will begin with chemotherapy using Adriamycin and Cytoxan, followed by radiation and then additional chemotherapy with Taxol." He took some time to explain the regimen and answer our questions, and while my initial apprehension waned, it was replaced in part with the sadness of realizing what Muriel is to endure. Luckily, this passed almost immediately due to the first words out of Muriel's mouth: "Will my treatment impact our travel plans?"

Dr. Koenig chuckled a bit and her spirit elicited a smile from me as well. "We'll work around your travels as best we can." We continued to discuss our plans in more detail and the air of fear and despair that had pervaded my thoughts was forgotten for a moment.

"We're going to Smugglers' Notch in Vermont in December, and then Texas right after Christmas," she said. "And then we're heading to British Columbia a few weeks after that."

Dr. Koenig reiterated his desire to do his best to work with our schedule, but by then I was thinking more about skiing and family visits and our lives than about chemotherapy and radiation. Muriel's peace was indeed contagious, and watching her soar above this storm, as she was doing here before my eyes in the face of what was by all measures a life-altering event, was a remarkable thing to behold. I was flying with her, and again I felt as though we had been blessed.

Dr. Koenig must have caught the feeling too as before long he had moved on to Muriel's future prospects. "If you remain cancer-free for five years, having cancer after that would be due to a new cancer and not a result of the breast cancer." He reviewed her list of medications and asked her to no longer take the Prempro. As far as all of the other medications on her list, she was free to continue taking them.

Toward the end of our appointment, Dr. Koenig described the next steps. "I want you to have an X-ray, a bone scan, a MUGA scan, and a CT scan. This will establish a baseline set of pictures of the internal organs of your body. If any changes occur in the future, as evidenced by updated pictures, the baseline pictures will assist in the prognosis."

Lastly, Muriel shared one of her vulnerabilities, though in retrospect I suppose this too was part of "normal" for us considering how long she had lived with it. "I have this great phobia about having needles stuck into my body."

Dr. Koenig had an answer for this as well. "We'll have Dr. Flynn surgically put in a port. Then you'll be able to have blood drawn easily and it will help you to avoid setting up an IV line each time you have chemotherapy."

We thought that sounded like a great idea and again a high note was struck. Dr. Koenig told us he looked forward to working with us and directed us to have his staff set up appointments for the different scans that Muriel was to have. We met with Laura again who explained all about the chemotherapy that Muriel would have and its effects: the nausea, the loss of hair, and the general malaise associated with the introduction of those chemicals into her body.

She then outlined the schedule of the chemotherapy sessions, taking into account the travel schedule we had planned and affording Muriel another opportunity to talk about the great things we would be doing. Laura also gave us some information about the radiation therapy that would follow the initial chemotherapy and several journals from the American Cancer Society that would provide answers to frequently asked questions. We seemed to be overwhelmed with information, but in a good way. The latent fear that I had felt earlier had already long subsided, but now I was overcome with an overpowering feeling of hope as we experienced all of the care and commitment of Dr. Koenig and his staff.

Muriel took a seat in the waiting room while I worked with the staff contact person to establish appointments for the three scans requested by Dr. Koenig. With that accomplished we went up one floor to Dr. Flynn's office to set up an appointment to have a port put in. Fortunately for us he had an opening the following morning to which we agreed. From there we went to the outpatient laboratory at City Hospital where Muriel had her X-ray.

It was after noontime when we finally arrived home. We ate lunch and discussed the events of the morning. Muriel well summed it up saying, "We will do what has to be done." And at that moment, and long thereafter, we both knew that we would. The peace of God had enveloped her, and I was there to support and help her in any way that I could to make her adventure as easy as possible. I thanked God again, this time for the inspiration we were feeling.

In the afternoon we held some interviews of fellow members of our Redeemer congregation to gather information for a database we are trying to establish at church. Those members we visited were equally amazed at Muriel's resilience and willingness to do this work in light of what she was still scheduled to endure. At day's end, my evening prayers were as positive and optimistic as I had offered since Muriel's adventure, our adventure, had begun, and sleep came easily.

Thursday, October 22, 1998

It was back to the hospital again today where Muriel had a port put in so that she can have chemotherapy and blood draws without the search for a vein each time she came in. It was placed under the skin just above her heart and connected to a small vein. It was completed as outpatient surgery and we were soon on our way.

We completed two more interviews for our church database and in the evening we had Stephen Ministry supervision. Supervision is basically a session of all Stephen Ministers where we meet for support and guidance from one another as we share the experiences with our various care receivers, with great emphasis placed on maintaining the anonymity of the individual care receivers. It was another busy day and Muriel continues to amaze me as well as others with her stamina, considering it is just three days short of one month since she had her initial surgery.

Friday, October 23, 1998

As is typical in life, some days are better than others, Muriel's adventure being no exception. Today we made another trip to the hospital where Muriel had the bone scan. Because of the difficulty Muriel experiences when she has to have a blood draw or a needle put in for an IV, I always accompany her into the room where the work is to be done. The technician told me I could not come into the room, but I was not about to let Muriel go in there by herself. I politely insisted that Muriel needed me to be with her and fortunately for us the technician yielded.

Unfortunately, because of the newness of the port that had just been put in yesterday, it could not be used. If not for this Muriel would not have had to endure the difficulties she encountered. I don't know if my presence upset the technician, but it turned out to be a worse-than-usual experience for Muriel. Initially the technician had a problem finding a vein in the arm but finally got an IV established, but then proceeded to dislodge the needle as she was in the process of securing it for use and had to start all over again. Muriel was in tears by the time this process was completed, and the technician provided us some time together before the scan began.

We were scheduled to go out to dinner in the evening and then to the concert by the Cleveland Orchestra at Severance Hall. However, after Muriel's ordeal with the bone scan we decided to not make the trip to Cleveland. We enjoyed a simple dinner at home and Muriel did at least find a silver lining at the tail end of the day. "At least we'll be able to use the port next time."

Sunday, October 25, 1998

We attended church today and then after lunch we hiked trail number nine. We both felt like taking it a bit easy so we decided to hike a trail that had a level of difficulty of one which we completed without any problems. Today marked the one-month anniversary of Muriel's original surgery. During that time she has received many cards from friends at church, friends at work, and other friends made through Marriage Encounter where we together served as a presenting couple for several years. Each card seems to bolster her, and she always makes it a point to write a thank you card or note to the person or persons who had sent the card. Many of the people receiving a response card from Muriel shared that they in turn were bolstered by her note of appreciation.

Two persons in our congregation, Donna Thrush, whose husband had died of cancer, and Betty Dodd, who was a breast cancer survivor, are very faithful with their card ministry. They always seem to arrive at a time when a bolstering is needed. It is amazing to me what a card with a handwritten note can do to one's spirits on any given day. *I'm thinking of you.* A simple gesture perhaps, yet so powerful, uplifting, and yet another reason we felt blessed.

Monday, October 26, 1998

It was back to the hospital today for a MUGA scan. I went to the examination room with Muriel while she got prepped. I was then requested to leave while the examination was in progress. The test was completed in a little over an hour and afterwards we stopped at Dick's Sporting Goods where I was in the market for ski wear. I tried on a pair of ski pants, a Columbia ski jacket with a liner, and ski gloves. We left the store with all of these new items, setting me up for many warmly dressed skiing forays for years to come.

Thursday, October 29, 1998

This morning Muriel had a CT scan scheduled for 8:30. Again I accompanied her into the examination room and held her hand while they put in an IV. I then retired to the waiting room while the test was completed.

From there we went to the outpatient laboratory where Muriel had an X-ray. By the time all of this activity was completed it was approaching noontime and we walked across the street to the Country Kitchen where we had lunch. We returned to our home at 87 Oakhurst Drive and settled in to watch one of Muriel's videos.

"Pick a letter," Muriel said, initiating a game we often played.

"S for sweetheart."

And in moments we had decided on that "feel good" gem *Sleepless in Seattle*. All of Muriel's 600 videos were displayed in a specially-built wall case in our family room, a monument to Muriel's unparalleled organization, though her sister termed it being "anal retentive." Whatever the label, I called it amazing, and it sure made our lives a lot less chaotic.

Her collection is a mix of purchased tapes and those she has taped herself from television. All of the tapes are neatly labeled and arranged in alphabetical order. When new ones arrive it is necessary to shift tapes and she generally waits until she has six or seven new tapes before integrating them among the old ones.

Then there is the listing we had just consulted, the ever-evolving Klafehn movie guide. It is an archive of our film library that Muriel has created on the computer, complete with the alphabetical listing of titles, the main stars, the length of the tape, where she got it, and even the cost for those she bought. Periodically she will print out a complete listing which is kept in a binder in the family room for quick consultation. She made similar listings of all of our CDs and cassette tapes. Yes, perhaps anal retentive fits the bill, but to me it was just another reason to love her and appreciate the order she brought to our lives. Her organizational skills were indeed a gift from the Lord.

Friday, October 30, 1998

Naked came I out of my mother's womb, and naked shall I return thither: the Lord gave, and the Lord hath taken away; blessed be the name of the Lord. Job 1:21.

We went to a funeral today at our church. A service was held for Peg Potter, one of our members, who had died from the complications of cancer. From what I have heard it is said that everyone has a relative, or a friend at work or in church, who has died from cancer. I hadn't really thought too much about it until cancer entered our own little world. I am beginning to fully fathom that statement.

Muriel was given a prosthesis the first time she visited Dr. Flynn's office after the operation and has been wearing it off and on ever since, more off than on. She finds it to be uncomfortable and always seems to be shifting in her bra, which increases the discomfort. She was never happy about wearing a bra when she had two breasts and would often remove it as soon as we entered the house, sometimes even removing it when we got into the car. How she could slip the strap down one arm and over the hand with a blouse on, and then pull the bra out the sleeve of the other arm, had always amazed me. She decided to wear the prosthesis today when we went to dinner at the Tavern on the Square where we enjoyed the extensive salad bar. I had prime rib for a main course with baked potato and steamed vegetables, and Muriel had grilled grouper with rice pilaf and steamed vegetables. We were stuffed after that and had no dessert. We did enjoy a cup of coffee before moving on to E. J. Thomas Hall where we had tickets for a night of Celtic music with Maura O'Connell and Solas. It was a delightful program and ranked right up there with Nightnoise and other *Thistle & Shamrock* offerings.

Saturday, October 31, 1998

Today is my birthday and I was the recipient of the family birthday card. It was several years ago while enjoying one of our time-share weeks in Tennessee that we had ventured into a local pharmacy to browse. At times like that we always check out the cards they have and pick out different cards for each other and say, "If I were to buy you a card today this is what I would get." Then we would exchange them and enjoy the sentiment or the humor of the selected card. It was a fun game we enjoyed playing. It was on this day that we found what has become our joint birthday card. The sentiment that it conveys is just how we feel about each other. It is a trifold design printed on a heavy card stock. There are orange and yellow orchids with green stems and yellowish backgrounds around the flowers. The words are written in cursive and at the beginning and end the words are three times the size of the rest of the lettering on the card. Below I have conveyed the sentiment of the card:

I love you.

I love being with you,
not only on your birthday,
but all the time.

I love all the joy that having you near can bring,
from our most intimate moments alone
to the pride I feel when we're out somewhere together.

I love all that we share.
I love the laughter,
the understanding,
and the fact that
so much about us—
our minds, our bodies,
our hearts, our feelings—
should touch so closely
and perfectly together.

Most of all, I love you,
and the gentle person you are with me—
the sensitive and loving side you save just for me
when we're alone together.

Happy Birthday,
with all my love.

Each time the card is conveyed, the date of the birthday is affixed to the back of the card and the card is retained by the recipient until it is time to pass it on to the other.

Muriel made me a special dinner called Saucy Sausage Skillet. It is a pasta dish made with ziti, cauliflower, broccoli, and turkey kielbasa with a Swiss and Monterey Jack cheese sauce. Parmesan cheese and pimentos were also added to the sauce. We had a nice White Zinfandel wine and a dessert of pecan pie. I am now 64 years old. I continue to be amazed at the way Muriel has accepted all that has taken place in her life thus far. She continues to be very positive, which I take as evidence of the peace from God that she had prayed for and received.

Monday, November 2, 1998

Today I had occasion to call United Airlines to change flight plans we had made. In the course of the conversation that I had with the customer service representative I shared that Muriel had breast cancer and had had a radical mastectomy of the right breast. As it turned out the representative also had had breast cancer including a mastectomy. She suggested that Muriel go to a health food store and stock up on CoQ10, Echinacea, and other health remedies which may ease the discomfort of chemotherapy as well as bolster her immune system.

I shared all of this with Muriel and she agreed to go to New Earth, a health food store in our area, to find out what she could about natural remedies. After lunch Muriel had an appointment to see Dr. Flynn. He wanted to check on the port which had been implanted. He judged that all was healing well but he wanted her to have another chest X-ray to see if there was anything under the skin that was improper. From his office we went to the outpatient X-ray lab.

Tuesday, November 3, 1998

Since today is the first Tuesday after the first Monday in November it was voting day and we stopped off at our local precinct on our way to Dr. Koenig's office where Muriel was to have her first chemotherapy session. Her appointment was scheduled for 10:00 and we arrived at about 9:45. Patty came for us at 10:00 and Muriel was weighed and taken to an examination room. Dr. Koenig examined her incision and talked about the chemotherapy she would be having.

"The chemotherapy will aggressively attack the cancer and weaken your immune system," he said, "so you'll need to have your white blood cell count monitored regularly. If the count is too low you'll need to wait until it increases to the acceptable range to have chemotherapy."

From the examination area Muriel was taken to the chemotherapy room, a long, narrow room approximately 20 feet by 12 feet that had six chairs. Five of them had their backs to the windows on the long side of the room. The sixth chair was facing the other chairs and was tucked back into an alcove. It was the one Muriel selected as it was the only seat unoccupied. There was a metal bookcase to the immediate right as you entered the room. It contained a small television, pillows, and books and magazines for the benefit of the patients receiving chemotherapy. On the left was a refrigerator containing soda and juices for the patients or those accompanying a patient. It also contained the chemotherapy mixtures that had been prepared in the Ritzman Pharmacy and walked over to the office in a refrigerated container. There was a counter on the other long wall with many cabinets both above and below the counter, where the nurses did their work.

The other five chairs were filled with individuals in various stages of receiving chemotherapy and were involved in a give-and-take with the nurses and other individuals having chemo. Some of the people had someone with them, others were by themselves. Some of them were reading as IVs continued their incessant drip. As we came into the room Patty said, "This is Muriel, who will begin her first treatment today." We were welcomed into the fold of camaraderie.

Muriel now experienced the beauty of having had a port put in. Prior to leaving home she had put a small dab of EMLA cream, a numbing salve, on the skin at the site of the port. The nurse then just pushed the needle into the port. No pain. No problems. Initially the line was cleared with a saline drip and then a vial of blood was drawn for testing. The white blood cell count was 7.7, within the acceptable range of 4.8 to 10.8.

The chemo bags, one with 92 mg of Adriamycin and the other with 920 mg of Cytoxan, were hung on the IV pole and the process began. The drip was regulated to take approximately 90 minutes for all of the "Kool-Aid," as it was referred to, to be filtrated into her body. We both had brought something to read. I sat on a stool beside her chair. We held hands and periodically read as we shared this new experience. At the end she was given an intravenous shot of 20 mg of Zofran and 12 mg of Decadron. Then the line was cleared with another saline drip and the first chemotherapy session was complete. We said goodbye to everyone and headed for home. We had been told many times about the side effects of chemotherapy, but Muriel experienced none of the nausea that was often present in others.

On the drive home Muriel said, "I'll be losing my hair soon. Do you think I should get a wig or just buy a bunch of hats?"

I was a bit biased since I had been shaving my head since 1973. "Why not go bald like me and wear a hat when necessary?"

"That sounds like a good idea but I still want to look at wigs and see how I would look in one."

I nodded and tried to visualize Muriel wearing a wig. I think at the time it was easier than imagining her without hair. Dr. Koenig sent Muriel home with three prescriptions, so we stopped at the pharmacy on the way home to drop them off. Two of them were of the pill variety, Zofran, 8 mg, and Torecan, 10 mg, and the third was a suppository, Phenergan, 25 mg. I went back later in the day to pick them up as Muriel pretty much cooled it for the rest of the day. I made Chicken Divan for dinner. Broccoli is one of Muriel's favorite vegetables so she ate heartily. She took one of the pills when she went to bed. She had not complained of any nausea but decided to take one as a preventative measure.

Wednesday, November 4, 1998

We both went for a flu shot at 10:00 this morning. Since we were concerned that the chemotherapy would be attacking Muriel's immune system, she had gotten approval to have the flu shot. Every preventative measure is to be taken. I ran several errands during the remainder of the day while Muriel curled up in her La-Z-Boy recliner with a book. We had leftovers from the previous night for dinner and then at 7:00 we went to bell choir practice. I have observed no ill effects in her from the chemotherapy thus far. In fact, with the exception of the one pill she took last night, she took none of the prescription drugs she had gotten as she did not experience any nausea.

Thursday, November 5, 1998

Today we drove to New Earth as Muriel wanted to investigate some of the natural drugs that might be beneficial to her immune system at this time. The sales assistant we encountered at the store was Sue Wells. As it turned out Sue was a breast cancer survivor, and after we explained our reason for being there she took Muriel in hand and made several suggestions. We started with Greens & More, and IP-6, both of which were enhancers to the immune system. The latter was a pill taken with water and the Greens & More was a powder which was mixed with water and then drunk. We also picked up a bottle of CoQ10 which was to be taken to protect her heart.

Of course Muriel and Sue shared about their common experience. Because there had been several individuals who had come into the store with similar circumstances, Sue was anticipating starting a support group that would meet monthly, and added Muriel's name to her list of potential participants. When we departed Muriel was rather excited to know that a support group was being formed. She is looking forward to being part of it.

Friday, November 6, 1998

We went out to dinner at Applebee's where I had the tilapia with mango salsa and Muriel had the lemon chicken. We both had a garden fresh salad and we shared a hot fudge sundae for dessert. After dinner we were off to the ballet. Muriel is now three days removed from her first chemotherapy session but amazingly she appears to suffer absolutely no ill effects.

Sunday, November 8, 1998

We went to both church services today. Muriel and I tended to flip-flop the service we attended because Communion is offered at the first service on the first and third Sundays of the month, and at the second service on the second and fourth Sundays, so we would go to the service where we could take Communion. This Sunday the bell choir was scheduled to play for the 8:15 service and Communion was scheduled for the second service. We went to Bible class in between the services and then we went to a kickoff luncheon for the Akron Symphony Orchestra. They were in the process of having a fund drive to increase the endowment for the orchestra. It was a full morning and early afternoon so Muriel was happy to get back home and curl up in her La-Z-Boy.

Tuesday, November 10, 1998

A very busy day. We had Stephen Ministry supervision at 11:00 in the morning. Many of our Stephen Ministers are retired so it is logical to meet during the day rather than take another night out of the week. In the afternoon Muriel was scheduled to meet with Dr. Flynn so he could take a look at the port he had put in. All was well. From his office we went to Dr. Koenig's office where Muriel had a blood test to check on her white blood cell count. The white blood cell (WBC) count was at 4.2, slightly below the normal range, the red blood cell (RBC) count was 4.51, about midway in the acceptable range, and the platelets level was 342, slightly above the preferred range, but apparently none of them critical.

As a result we celebrated by going out to dinner at The Olive Garden in the Chapel Hill Mall. We devoured the big bowl of salad and ate the breadsticks. Muriel had a pasta primavera and I had pork chops with an Alfredo sauce. We each enjoyed a glass of Chardonnay with our meal and decided to forgo dessert. After dinner we had Chorale practice and then bell choir. It was past 9:00 when we got home. It was another jam-packed day and Muriel continues to do well.

Friday, November 13, 1998

"Friday the 13th falls on a Friday this month," Muriel joked.

I laughed. "Yes it does." Of course she would say that regardless of the day of the week it fell on, always eliciting a smile from me. She continues to amaze me with her energy and stamina. We did some cleaning in the house and Muriel did some wash and a little ironing. In the evening we drove to Cleveland and had dinner at a favorite Chinese restaurant on Cedar Road. When Muriel broke open her fortune cookie she stared in amazement and shared the statement with me, "A new adventure begins with a single step."

After dinner we were on to Severance Hall and a Cleveland Orchestra concert. Jahja Ling was the conductor for the evening and the first half of the program was a viola concerto by Gubaidulina featuring Yuri Bashmet as the guest violist. The second half of the program was the Tenth Symphony by Shostakovich, who is not one of our favorite composers, so we decided not to stay and headed home early. Our return home wasn't quite as late as was typical for a Cleveland Orchestra concert and we were happy for that.

Monday, November 16, 1998

I made a trip to the Metro Parks office in the morning to bring in our hiking forms and pick up our medallions for the '98 Fall Hiking Spree. From there I went to C. L. Davis, a jeweler in downtown Akron. I had a double purpose in mind: one was to find an eagle pin, emblematic of soaring above the clouds, and the second was to have a pendant with an etching of the words "Soaring Above the Clouds." I intended to give Muriel the pendant as soon as it was ready and the eagle was to be a Christmas present. All of the pins that he had at the store were of eagles with wings spread and talons down which was not the type that I was looking for. The jeweler had several catalogs available so I looked through them and discovered an eagle that appealed to me. I ordered it and was home by lunchtime.

After lunch we went to a Hudson hair salon where the owner maintained wigs for individuals who were going through chemotherapy and had suffered the temporary loss of hair. Muriel has always had naturally curly hair and I had never seen her in curlers. She could just shower, brush the snags out, set a few finger waves, and be set to go. She has always worn her hair short and in fact, we had gotten to a point where I was allowed to cut it. So Muriel was not exactly ecstatic about getting a wig. She tried on several different styles and seemed to be dissatisfied with each of them. Her comment was always, "They make me look like I'm wearing a wig." I was not about to make a comment on that statement, though I thought she looked nice in two of the styles.

She decided to not get a wig at this time, and instead wanted to look through some of the catalogs she had at home and perhaps order several hats. Several turned out to be an understatement as I think all told she ended up with about 15 different hats before she was done. Later on she even came home with a wig, though I think I wore it more than she did. Given my beard, when I wore the wig she'd say, "You look like Kris Kristofferson!" However, I think I only wore it out of the house once when we went to a church get-together. Since I normally shave my head, it is amazing what a head of hair can do for one's appearance. Initially there were very few people who recognized me and wondered who Muriel had brought with her. Often, on very cold nights, I would wear it to bed to keep my head warm.

Tuesday, November 17, 1998

Back to Arch Street today and Dr. Koenig's office where Muriel had a blood test. Once again the WBC count was 1.9, below the acceptable range but not a critical figure. The RBC count was 4.15 and the platelets were 342. The use of the port is paying big dividends as far as Muriel's comfort is concerned. A little numbing cream on the surface and there was no feeling at all when she experienced the needle prick.

Friday, November 20, 1998

Today marks eight weeks since Muriel had her initial operation. She has had one chemotherapy session with absolutely minimal side effects. The two blood tests she has had indicated a WBC count that is slightly below the acceptable range but again, not critical. Her energy level is very normal. People at church ask me how I am doing and it is easy to be very upbeat because of Muriel's faith and attitude toward her adventure. She enjoys sleeping in in the morning so I tiptoe around so as to not disturb her. She has regularly done the washing and ironing as well as most of the cooking. Sometimes on Sundays I will make brunch or dinner, and maybe even one of the planned meals during the week. As strange as it may sound, things are pretty much back to normal.

Our daughter Kay invited us out to Texas and ultimately Pagosa Springs, Colorado where she and her family planned to go skiing at Wolf Creek Ski Resort for the Thanksgiving holiday. Muriel was reluctant to go but encouraged me to go and ski with Kay and her family. I refused initially, skeptical about going and leaving Muriel behind during the holiday, but as usual she was insistent that I go.

I again realized my blessings and began making plans to fly to Denver where I would rent a car and drive to Salida, Colorado to spend a night with my sister Karen. I would then drive down to Wolf Creek to meet up with Kay and her family. I was excited about skiing, as I had just learned this past spring when Kay had invited us to Angel Fire in New Mexico. I had taken a group ski lesson in the morning and another in the afternoon and I was hooked.

This afternoon Muriel and I went to C. L. Davis, the jewelry store, to pick up her pendant only to discover that I had them etch "Soaring Above the Clouds," when it should have been "Soaring Above the Storm." The jeweler indicated that the surface was thick enough for him to be able to polish the surface and re-etch the proper wording back onto the surface. On our return home we stopped at the Finast grocery store to pick up a few special grocery items for Muriel's home stay.

Saturday, November 21, 1998

Today was a typical Saturday. I stripped the beds and washed and dried the sheets and remade the beds. I made a batch of Date Nut Oaties, our favorite cookie. This way Muriel would have some munchies while I was away. We went out to dinner at the Macaroni Grill and then to an Akron Symphony Orchestra concert. Betsy Burleigh, who is the regular director of the Akron Symphony Chorus, directed all of the pieces this evening. The first piece on the program was Beethoven's Mass in C Major, Op. 78, featuring the Akron Symphony Chorus. The second piece was Symphony No. 3 in C Minor, Op. 78 by Saint-Saëns. It was an organ concerto featuring Richard Shirey, a member of the music department at the University of Akron. The combined effort of the orchestra and chorus on the C Major Mass was superb, and adding in the organ concerto made it feel almost like being in church. We departed the concert with an uplifted feeling that made for a gentle ride home.

Tuesday, November 24, 1998

Once again we began the day by driving into Akron so Muriel could have her blood tested. The WBC count was at 9.1, an elevation from last month and not a critical value—the higher number is good as long as it isn't too high. The RBC count was 4.3 and platelets were 436, above the upper range but not critical, so it looks like she will be able to have her next chemotherapy session. Muriel got a prescription for temazepam from Dr. Koenig which is designed to help in sleeping. I had taken my bag with me so we drove to the airport where Muriel dropped me off for my flight to Denver. Up until the last minute I hesitated about leaving her.

"Are you sure about this?"

"Absolutely," she assured me. "You go and have a good time. I know I'm going to."

"All right sweetheart. I'll be just a phone call away so please call me if you need anything."

"I will."

I kissed her goodbye and I was on my way. Muriel's "good time" plan was to spend Thanksgiving by herself and making one of her favorite meals, spaghetti with white clam sauce. She really was looking forward to it, but when people at church found out she was going to spend the holiday by herself she received several invitations for dinner. Muriel initially stuck with her original plan, but she did finally succumb to the pleadings and agreed to have dinner with Pastor Al and Barb Boehlke.

When I arrived in Denver, I called Muriel to let her know I had arrived safely and then I rented a car from Enterprise. The temperature was unseasonably warm, reaching the 70s, and as I drove down I-25 I could see people on the golf course. All I could think of was that I had left Muriel behind and it looked like I wasn't even going to be able to ski. However, as I drove into the mountains the temperature dropped and the prospects of skiing were greatly increased.

I finally reached Salida and met my sister Karen at the learning center where she tutored students who were deficient in reading skills. Karen is seven years younger than I, and I must admit that I picked on her mercilessly when we were growing up. However, in our adulthood we continue to be in touch, mainly through e-mail and other times when we have been able to get together through my traveling. She showed me around the center with its plethora of age-oriented books and then we drove to the ski shop that was operated by her friend John. I was fitted for boots and skis. John was very meticulous with my boots and took time to add lifts to complete the balancing. They felt absolutely great. After the boot fitting I took Karen out to dinner at a Chinese restaurant. Monarch Ski Resort is near Salida so the village is well equipped to handle the tourists from the East, including having a Chinese restaurant.

Wednesday, November 25, 1998

In the morning I continued on to Wolf Creek Ski Resort to meet my daughter and her family. I was standing in line to get my lift ticket when I heard, "Hi Grandpa." It was Kenton, Kay's 9-year-old son, greeting me. Kenton and I skied the morning together. "I like to ski with you Grandpa because when you get to the bottom you get right back on the lift and go back to the top." We went on to ski three of the four days we were there and then again on Sunday morning. Kay had brought a smoked turkey with all of the trimmings for Thanksgiving, as well as a ham. So if we were not eating a main meal of turkey or ham we were having sandwiches of turkey or ham. I enjoyed the trip immensely, especially the opportunity to see our daughter, her husband Larry, and our two grandchildren Kenton and Kaitlyn, who was 12. In the evenings we made popcorn and played Phase 10 or UNO. On Friday evening I called Muriel.

"Hello?"

"Hello, sweetheart. It's me."

"Wow, I didn't expect to hear from you. Did you take a spill?"

"No, I didn't take a spill. I just missed you and wanted to hear your voice. Plus I needed a break from Phase 10. Everybody except Larry is beating me."

"Oh, you poor baby."

"So how was your dinner at Pastor Al's?"

"I'll tell you all about it when you get home."

I retreated further from the Phase 10 activity and the next few minutes were just mine and Muriel's. I was relieved to hear how well she was doing.

"It *is* great to hear your voice," I said. "I've been praying for you every day and night."

"I know."

Before long, Kaitlyn approached asking, "Who are you speaking to Grandpa?"

"It's Oma. Sweetheart, your grandchildren want to talk to you."

The phone was handed to Kaitlyn, then Kenton, then Kay, and finally back to me.

"We plan on skiing in the morning and then I'll head for Salida to stay overnight with Karen. I look forward to seeing you on Monday. I love you."

"I love you too. Drive carefully."

Sunday, November 29, 1998

I did take a nasty spill this morning, skiing too fast and out of control. I landed hard on my chest. I thought perhaps I had broken a rib or two. It was uncomfortable breathing and really hurt if I took a deep breath or coughed. I was skiing with Larry and he assisted me to my feet and we skied to the bottom of the hill. I sat out the next couple of runs and a little after 1:00 I said goodbye to Kay, Larry, Kaitlyn, and Kenton and drove back to Salida.

I stopped at a gas station on my way and changed out of my ski clothes and into my jeans and a turtleneck sweater. When I reached Salida I asked my sister to direct me to the hospital. I wanted to have my hurting chest checked out. They performed all sorts of tests but indicated that nothing was broken. The diagnosis was a slight tear of the flesh away from the rib cage and that it would be painful for a while and then one morning it would be gone.

My sister had anticipated taking me to the health spa in Salida. The facility is fed by natural springs, so there are pools where the temperature is 102 degrees and varying lesser degrees in other pools. The warmth felt great on my aching ribs. It was difficult to swim so I just lulled in the pool. Kay had sent me on my way with leftover turkey and ham plus other goodies, so Karen and I had a second Thanksgiving dinner. I stayed the night with my sister and we reminisced about living at our childhood home and enjoying the holidays. After we had cleaned up from dinner Karen asked, "How is Muriel doing?"

"Initially, I was reluctant to even come on this trip, but she insisted. Her adventure, as she terms it, is running on all cylinders. At the time of her diagnosis, she told me she prayed for peace and God provided it instantly and she has been on a roll ever since."

"Has she started chemotherapy yet?"

"Yes, she has had one session and would you believe, she had absolutely no side effects."

"It's amazing what God can do if you let Him."

"She will have her second session the day after I get back. Then comes radiation and then more chemotherapy."

"Well tell her she continues to be in my prayers."

"I will."

Monday, November 30, 1998

I woke up early feeling better but still sore. I said goodbye to Karen and headed to Denver. I turned in my rental car and got a boarding pass for my flight to Cleveland. I saw by the flight status board that there was an earlier flight to Cleveland so I asked to be put on standby for that. While I waited, I called Muriel.

"Good morning sweetheart. How are you?"

"I'm doing fine. How was the rest of your trip?" she asked.

She did still sound well and it was great to hear her voice again. I didn't want to burden her with news of my accident, so I decided to leave that out of our conversation for the moment.

"It was great, though I really missed you. Thank you for letting me come. I wish you could have come too."

"Me too, but I have to confess it has been nice and peaceful here. Just what the doctor ordered I suppose."

"That's great to hear but your respite might be shorter than you expected. I'm on standby for an earlier flight."

"That's fine by me. I'm looking forward to having you home."

"And I'm looking forward to seeing you. I'll call you if I'm lucky."

"Sounds good. Talk to you soon."

Armed with my usual *Sports Illustrated* I settled in to read and wait for my flight. Before long I was paged for the 10:20 flight and after exchanging my boarding pass I called Muriel to let her know I would be arriving earlier than anticipated. The flight was smooth and Muriel was there to pick me up, waiting in the baggage claim area of Cleveland Hopkins International Airport. I greeted her with a kiss and a hug. She looked great and even seemed to have added some color to her face.

We were eager to relate more of what had happened while we were apart, and talked as we drove to the Outback Steakhouse in Macedonia for a late lunch. After we were seated and had placed our order Muriel nonchalantly said, "I'm beginning to lose my hair." We had both anticipated this would likely happen, so I was not surprised at the news. Still, I fought back some of the emotion I felt at the revelation. She was wearing one of her new hats. It was of the style the Berenstain Bears wear, so all the hats of that style got the generic assignment of Berenstain Bear hats.

We didn't dwell on her hair and chatted all through lunch, she about her Thanksgiving dinner with the Boelhkes and I about my fall on the mountain and about our daughter and her family. But my mind often returned to thoughts of the changes Muriel was undergoing from her adventure. I was amazed at how well she had adjusted thus far. When we got home she had me use the electric clippers on her hair. I put a number three rake on the clippers and proceeded to cut it all to a height of about three-eighths of an inch. We now begin a new phase in our togetherness, both of us without hair.

Tuesday, December 1, 1998

This morning we were on our way to Dr. Koenig's office for Muriel's second chemotherapy session. This was another reason Muriel had decided not to go to Colorado, as she would be having chemotherapy the day after we returned and thought she might be pushing it. She initially had a blood draw and the WBC count was 10.1, within the acceptable range. The RBC count was 4.44 and platelets were at 380. She next was routinely examined by Dr. Koenig. Muriel shared her non-reaction to her first round of chemotherapy.

"That's great to hear," he said, "but don't be surprised if that changes as we move forward." He provided her with another prescription for the EMLA cream and then she proceeded to the chemotherapy room where she took her place in the corner chair in the alcove. Three of the patients in the room had been there the last time. The "Kool-Aid" cocktail was the usual Adriamycin and Cytoxan. One of the other people receiving chemo was a real character and had us laughing much of the time, the laughter a medicine unto itself. The 90 minutes passed by quickly and it was soon time for the saline drip. Muriel seemed somewhat subdued when we departed but claimed she felt fine.

On the way home we stopped at C. L. Davis and picked up her pendant which now properly read, "Soaring Above the Storm." She seemed to be greatly uplifted by the pendant and immediately put it on. I got her home and made her a grilled cheese sandwich for lunch and settled her into her La-Z-Boy while I went out to work in the backyard. We have a feral backyard and I have been trying to clean it up since I had retired. We were enjoying a spell of warm weather and I felt obligated to get it cleaned up as best I could. Mind you it was not one of my favorite things to do, but I just kept plugging away. It had to be done some time, after all we have only lived there since 1974! My philosophy had always been, if the weather was nice enough to work in the backyard then it was nice enough to play golf. So I generally went and played golf, often with Muriel.

But today the backyard beckoned me, or was it taunting me? Either way, I sought to spend some time today restoring order to it. I am sure that Muriel's remarkably balanced approach to her adventure has elevated me as well. Her God-given ability to maintain order in the face of what could have been a tremendous upheaval of our lives, her soaring, sailing, even smiling above the storm, inspires me to do things that have long caused anxiety.

Thursday, December 3, 1998

We shopped today at the Finast grocery store buying all the items necessary for our sustenance for the month. The list of menu items was not too long as we had made plans to travel several of the days of the month, but list highlights included some of the ingredients we would need to prepare our traditional Christmas fare, something we both looked forward to enjoying on Christmas Eve.

As one can see by the date of this shopping trip, we didn't always shop on the first of the month. Because of Muriel's process and us dining out unexpectedly we sometimes had meals left over at the end of the month and those would carry us into the beginning of the following month. Her planning served us well again today.

Friday, December 4, 1998

Muriel was getting low on some of the herbal palliatives that she was taking so we went to New Earth to buy those items as well as some antioxidants that she needed. She was able to visit with her friend Sue Wells and was introduced to another breast cancer survivor, Robin Graham. Plans are still in the making for the support group and Sue indicated that it will probably come together in the new year.

Since we were leaving on our next vacation the following day, we spent the rest of the morning and afternoon packing. In the evening we drove to Cleveland where we ate dinner at the China Gate Restaurant in Cleveland Heights and then went to the Cleveland Orchestra concert at Severance Hall. Christian Thielemann was the guest conductor and the orchestra performed "Night Scene in the Park" by Siegfried Matthus and Mozart's Piano Concerto No. 20, K. 466, with Leif Ove Andsnes as the piano soloist. The second half of the program was Beethoven's Fifth Symphony which sent everyone home very uplifted. Even though it was another late night and Muriel is three days removed from her last chemotherapy session, she was in a great mood and very upbeat. God truly answers prayers. The peace that she had prayed for is still working wonders.

Saturday, December 5, 1998

Today we embarked on another time-share trip. I was somewhat unsure, not being familiar with MapQuest at the time, how long it would take us to drive to Smugglers' Notch in Vermont so our plan was to drive as far as the Albany, New York area and then stay overnight.

We left at 6:30 in the morning and drove on I-80 across Pennsylvania, and then took I-81 north to the New York State Thruway, I-90. This brought us into Albany and we stopped at a Red Roof Inn in Colonie, New York. We had dinner at Denny's and then went back to the motel to relax and get some sleep.

Sunday, December 6, 1998

We were up early and went to Denny's for breakfast. We encountered all of the Sunday morning churchgoers having their breakfasts as well, though we decided to wait and luckily were soon seated. We both had the Grand Slam breakfast. It always amazes me in that Muriel never eats breakfast when we are home but always eats breakfast when we travel. Who can figure it out? We were finally headed to Smugglers' Notch in Vermont by 9:00. Our trip took us through Burlington and Essex Junction, finally arriving midafternoon at Smugglers' Notch. The condo was probably less than a year old and was just gorgeous. We unpacked and I watched the late football games. The prospect of skiing looks bleak, but who knows what tomorrow will bring?

Sunday, December 13, 1998

We returned to Munroe Falls today, making the whole journey home in one day. As was generally the case, Muriel and I took turns driving, with each of us behind the wheel two to three hours at a stretch. Our week came during the impeachment trial of President Bill Clinton so that occupied some of our time. I never did get to ski, but we had a great time relaxing and exploring the region. We drove over to Stowe and checked out all of the little shops. We bundled up and went for several walks, checking out the ski shop and other shops in the area. Muriel had brought along her usual quota of seven books and slowly worked her way through them. I too had brought some books but I interspersed my reading time with the completion of a 1,000-piece jigsaw puzzle. In addition, they had a heated outdoor swimming pool where the water temperature was 85 degrees. I swam a couple of times but it was nasty getting from the changing area to the pool and back. While swimming, I tried to stay underwater as much as I could as the outside temperature was in the 20s. Even though Muriel had just completed her second chemotherapy session she looked and felt great the entire trip.

Tuesday, December 15, 1998

We left for Dr. Koenig's office so Muriel could have her blood checked. The WBC count was 2.2 which was below the acceptable range. The RBC count was 3.79, also below the preferred range. However, the platelets count was at 297 which did fall in the acceptable range. Apparently there was nothing critical as we were sent on our way. We stopped at Mister Bulky on the way home to pick up the rest of the supplies we would need to make treats for the Christmas season, in particular some walnuts, dates, and carob so I can make cookies.

In the evening we went to Chorale practice where we reviewed the numbers we are scheduled to sing on Christmas Eve. Tonight was the unveiling of Muriel's nearly bald head at Chorale practice. Appropriate comments about us now being twins were bandied about with everyone having a good-natured laugh at Muriel's expense. However, she was unfazed by it all.

Tuesday, December 22, 1998

We said a prayer for our son, Mark, this morning as today is his 39th birthday. Chemotherapy session number three was scheduled for today, so I inwardly prayed that all would continue to go well. As Muriel has progressed through her treatment there seems to be a certain resignation, like *point me in the right direction and let's get on with it*. There is not a negative demeanor in her manner but simply the attitude *I'll do what I have to do so I can get on with my life*. The usual routine was undertaken in Dr. Koenig's office. Get weighed, have her blood pressure taken, get examined, and then into the chemo room.

Each time Muriel has had chemotherapy she expresses her happiness at having a port so the search for a vein does not have to take place. Two members of the chemotherapy group had completed their cycle so we had two new additions to the group. Mr. Humor was still among us and helped keep the atmosphere light. Nurse Pattie got Muriel hooked up to the IV. Initially there was the saline flush and then a blood draw. Her blood counts were within the acceptable range and she proceeded with her session. The filtration of the Adriamycin and Cytoxan took approximately 90 minutes and then there was another saline drip. As we departed, Muriel expressed how great she felt so we stopped at Applebee's at the Chapel Hill Mall and had lunch. She relaxed when we got home and I made two batches of cookies, Date Nut Oaties and Magic Cookie Bars. We both agreed that they passed the pre-Christmas Eve taste test.

Wednesday, December 23, 1998

We worked around the house in the morning in preparation for our trip to Texas to see our children and grandchildren. Our plan was to start our drive early on Christmas Day, which would be a bit of a challenge given our plans for Christmas Eve. After lunch we took in the matinee theater and saw *Notting Hill* with Hugh Grant and Julia Roberts, another of those "feel good" movies, we, especially Muriel, were fond of. Since the movie was at the Plaza 8 at Chapel Hill we spontaneously stopped off at Mario's Eastside Restaurant and had dinner, one of the unplanned meals out that would leave us with another meal left over for the beginning of January. Planned or not, it was a welcome occasion as Mario's specializes in great Italian food. I decided to have their deluxe hamburger with fries and a big glass of Killian's Red. Muriel was more circumspect and had a grilled chicken sandwich, fries, and a glass of Killian's Red as well. Who said that nausea follows a chemotherapy session? The nausea that is so common for chemotherapy patients has thus far spared Muriel, a fortune for which we are both very grateful. The adventure continues.

Thursday, December 24, 1998

We went to the 10:00 p.m. candlelight service, primarily because the Chorale would be singing. We sang four different pieces, climaxing with a new number entitled, "Were You There?" It is a beautiful piece and is very appropriate for the Christmas season. We were able to share Communion together and arrived home at 11:30. We have had a tradition at Christmas time whereupon arriving home from church we have wine and snacks. The snacks consisted of shrimp, two kinds of cheese, Hickory Farms beef stick, homemade cheese ball, Triscuits, Wheat Thins, chips, and some of the cookies I had made. Muriel also made a spread that was put on party rye bread and then heated. So we snacked heartily as we opened presents. I gave Muriel her soaring eagle pin and symbolically, I placed the chain over her head that held the pendant that said "Soaring Above the Storm." The Chorale had given her a gift certificate to Borders bookstore. Just what we need, more books! The accompanist for the Chorale gave her a framed 5 by 7 picture of an eagle soaring through space. It was beautiful and was hung on the wall right next to her computer where she could see it each time she sat down to type. We finally headed for bed about 1:00, tired but content.

Friday, December 25, 1998

We were up at 4:00 a.m. and soon on our way to Texas. Muriel dressed for the trip the night before and spent the night in her La-Z-Boy. I on the other hand had spent what was left of the evening in the comfort of my bed. Our itinerary was to travel I-76 west to I-71, south to Columbus, and then take I-70 out of Columbus to the west. We crossed Indiana and made our way into Illinois, splitting off of I-70 just past Effingham and taking I-57 south to Cairo. We crossed the Mississippi River and eventually picked up I-55 south into Missouri.

If you have never traveled on Christmas Day, I suggest that you not even think about it. Admittedly there is little traffic, but hardly anything is open and, for all of our careful preparations, we hadn't planned for that. Fortunately we found a gas station that had sandwiches to go or we would never have eaten lunch. We drove south on I-55 as far as Blytheville, Arkansas and stayed the night at the Comfort Inn. We finally managed to find a take-out Chinese restaurant enabling us to enjoy dinner back in our room.

Saturday, December 26, 1998

We ate breakfast at McDonald's and then continued down I-55 to West Memphis where we turned west onto I-40 toward Little Rock. In Little Rock we took the loop and then got onto I-30 which would take us through Texarkana and right into Dallas. Muriel was driving as we passed through Greenville, Texas and encountered a reduced-speed construction zone. Apparently she did not slow down fast enough because we immediately had a Texas Highway Patrol car behind us with its lights flashing and its siren going. There was barely any room to pull off but Muriel managed to get the car up on the shoulder with the highway patrol pulling right in behind us.

First, it should be known that Muriel is a notorious "lead foot" when it came to driving. That is, until she got a speeding ticket in Arkansas a year or so earlier that had cost her $125.00. Since then she has set the cruise control at the posted speed and never deviated. That's why this stop by the Texas Highway Patrol was somewhat devastating since she had braked to disengage the cruise control and was in the process of slowing down, maintaining speed with the other traffic. The officer had no room to stand and talk on the driver's side, so he approached the car on the passenger side. He requested her license and registration. "Do you know how fast you were going through the construction area?"

Before she even answered I could sense the emotion building in her. "Yes, I was in the process of slowing down, and I, I was—" She paused, near tears, causing my own eyes to water, and reached for her hat, brandishing her bald head. She spoke swiftly and in one breath said, "I'm going through chemotherapy for cancer and I was doing my best and I always set the cruise control for the posted speed and I'm very conscious of the change in speed limits and try to drive accordingly. I'm truly sorry if I didn't slow down quickly enough."

I turned to the officer who glanced from Muriel to me and then back to Muriel again. Without a word and with just a simple nod, he stepped back to his car and in a moment was back at my window. He returned the license and registration and suggested she be careful of the speed limit and sent us on our way. I could be wrong but I am convinced that she was stopped because she was driving a car with out-of-state plates, because she was not going any faster than other cars with Texas plates. Regardless, the officer did at least let her go without citation, and we were thankful he allowed us to continue on our way.

At the next rest area we switched drivers and I continued on I-30 allowing Muriel to reduce her tension. I too relaxed a bit. We took the I-635 loop around the north perimeter of Dallas and headed up Preston Road to our daughter's house in Plano. We were both eager to see our new granddaughter, but Mark and his family were at his wife Cathy's parent's house in Llano, Texas for Christmas and would not be back until Sunday. Our plans were to spend a few days with Kay and her family, then move on to Mark's house in Flower Mound. Upon our arrival, the first thing was the unveiling of Muriel's bald head and the absorption of the comments that are attendant with that disclosure. Both of the kids had to rub her head and express the apparently universal joke that now Oma and Grandpa were twins. Muriel had a great relationship with our granddaughter Kaitlyn, helping her through a difficult time when her mother and father were divorced. She initially had a difficult time getting along with her stepfather Larry. Kenton has ADHD and has been a handful ever since he was born, but he is enrolled at a private school that is primarily for children like him and he is doing very well.

Thursday, December 31, 1998

Kay and Larry had season tickets to the Dallas Stars hockey games and yesterday Kay, Larry, Kenton and I were off to Reunion Arena to see the Dallas Stars play the Edmonton Oilers. Muriel remained at Kay's house to be with Kaitlyn. As today is New Year's Eve, Larry, a vice president of human resources for Brinker International, treated us to dinner at Maggiano's Little Italy where we had calamari and fried cheese sticks as appetizers, and for the entrée we had salmon and roast pork served family style. It was our second visit to this restaurant and the food was equally good. Afterward, we resumed the UNO and Phase 10 championship begun in Colorado.

43

Friday, January 1, 1999

We moved on to Mark's house and to Emma Catherine, the new baby, and of course the rest of her family. Muriel jumped at the chance to hold a brand new baby, at least new to her. Mark and Cathy also have another daughter, Meagan, who is ten. It is always nice to visit our children and grandchildren, but once you have an empty nest it is also nice to head back home and enjoy the peace and quiet of your own home. The world of teens and preteens passed us by some time ago.

Monday, January 4, 1999

We departed very early and stopped at McDonald's along I-30 in Greenville, Texas for breakfast. We generally have CDs playing as we drive, or we read to the driver or to ourselves, but today during my stints, I spent much of the time reflecting again on the way in which Muriel had handled all that had transpired. She still has one more chemotherapy session, and then radiation followed by more chemotherapy. As I thought about what was still to come, it seemed pretty daunting to me at first, but then I remembered, and marveled at, how well Muriel had done.

"I'm really proud of the way you have handled everything," I said.

"Thank you, but what choice is there really?" she asked. "We both have done what we have needed to do, and I don't see that changing in the future. But I'm proud of you too. We make a great team."

Bless her for her strength and inspiration. My mood was instantly elevated and the minutes passed quickly until she asked, "Should I have my left breast removed as a preventative measure?"

I didn't have an answer right then so she offered her thoughts on the idea. "If the breast did not exist there would be no chance of getting cancer in it." As I pondered her statement, she added, "And I will be better balanced too."

Finally I suggested, "Speak with all of the doctors you are seeing and get their collective opinions. They'll know better than I, so if it's something you want to consider we should consult with them."

She agreed, and that discomforting feeling crept back into my mind as it looked to me like the adventure was going to continue into another year. That feeling quickly subsided again though as I glanced over at Muriel who was peacefully gazing out the window, still at ease despite our discussion of another operation. We retraced our route out of Texas, finally arriving in Terre Haute, Indiana where we stayed at a Motel 6 and had dinner at the Red Lobster. We both slept soundly.

Tuesday, January 5, 1999

We completed our trip home to Munroe Falls and after we had unpacked, I picked up the newspapers and mail. We went to Applebee's for dinner and then dove right back into our active calendar by going to bell choir practice in the evening.

Wednesday, January 6, 1999

We went to Dr. Koenig's office so Muriel could have her blood drawn and analyzed. The WBC count was 2.9, on the low side of the range. The RBC count was 3.77 and the platelets count was 339, both in an acceptable range. So unless things change drastically Muriel is scheduled for her last chemotherapy session in one week.

Saturday, January 9, 1999

I kibitzed while Muriel prepared lasagna for our Chorale Christmas party which was to be held at Sonja Pusch's house. It was open to all Chorale members and their spouses. Sonja furnished many appetizers and "Glühwein," a warm wine of German origin. It is comprised of red wine, to which is added a cinnamon stick and other herbs to suit one's taste, all of which whetted our appetite for the main course, the lasagna that Muriel had made. Other members of the Chorale brought various dishes to complete our potluck fare. We had taken pictures of our newest granddaughter and shared them with those in attendance. Sonja's house was very festively decorated with a total of seven different Christmas trees upstairs and downstairs. Some were real, some were artificial, and all were spectacularly decorated.

Tuesday, January 12, 1999

Another trip to Dr. Koenig's office for the last dose of Adriamycin and Cytoxan. The office waiting area was crowded with cancer patients and those attending to them. I had thought often that the negative of a patient dying would weigh heavily on doctors who are cancer specialists, but apparently it is the survivors who provide the impetus for them to continue on in this specialized field. Muriel was weighed, had her blood pressure taken, and then was examined. After the examination Dr. Koenig outlined her progress and what was to come. "You have tolerated the chemotherapy very well. Today is the last session, with radiation therapy to follow. When that is done you'll return to complete the chemotherapy using Taxol and then we will begin the tamoxifen regimen." I again felt disheartened, but Muriel seemed at ease.

We moved from the examination room to the chemo room where Muriel found a chair just inside the door. Muriel's blood draw indicated a WBC count of 11.6, above the outer limit but not a critical value. The RBC count and the platelets were 3.86 and 675 respectively. We continued with the procedure. Once again Muriel suffered no ill effects from the chemotherapy so I raised up a prayer of thanksgiving. All of the nurses are impressed that she has had little or no nausea. The Lord's peace can apparently do wonders, though she did cool it for the rest of the day.

Thursday, January 14, 1999

Muriel and I went to New Earth again today to pick up more of the herbals that she is taking on a regular basis. She also had the opportunity to see her friend Sue Wells again and inquire about the support group. Robin Graham, who was also going through chemotherapy, was in the store as well and was sans hair just like Muriel. Robin too seemed excited about the support group and looked forward to its formation.

Sunday, January 24, 1999

Last Sunday we left on the last trip we had already scheduled before Muriel began her adventure. This past spring we had taken a cruise to the Eastern Caribbean and on our return to Cleveland, the Continental Airlines flight from Fort Lauderdale had been delayed for nearly twelve hours due to a faulty part on the plane. They had to fly a part in from Houston and then put it on the plane. We were given vouchers for lunch and then dinner as we waited at the airport, and finally we were sent on our way. We all also received a voucher worth $300.00 for use toward any flight on Continental at some future date in time. With Muriel's blessing I had scheduled another skiing trip, this time to Panorama in British Columbia.

What was interesting about the flight was the route we took. We flew out of Cleveland to Houston, and then to Calgary. That did not seem to be the most direct route to get there, but then I don't make the routes. Regardless, we arrived safely in Calgary where we rented a car for the drive to Panorama. We took Route 201 out of Calgary going west and on to Highway 1 west. The trip was uneventful, although you could see the Rockies in the distance, and as we continued our drive they loomed larger and larger. We turned south just beyond Banff onto Highway 93 and wound our way down through the mountains, merging with Highway 95. We exited the highway to take the final road to Panorama, but not before stopping at a grocery store in Invermere to buy groceries for the week.

Panorama is a self-contained resort with tons of snow in wintertime. We checked in and found we had underground parking. We unpacked and then went to the ski rental place so I could be fitted for boots and skis. The facility was adequate for our needs but was not as nice as the condos we had stayed in at Pagosa Springs and Smugglers' Notch. What was great, though, was the fact that I could walk out of the condo, step into my skis, and immediately get onto a ski lift. However, when you got to the top it was necessary to ski down to the lodge to buy a lift ticket. I signed up for a lesson later in the week and proceeded to try some of the slopes. Since there was a ski trail that led right back to the condo I returned at lunchtime to check on Muriel and have lunch.

Muriel, of course had brought along some books and was content to read while I skied. We walked in the afternoons, exploring the shops at the resort. We ate one of our meals at the local restaurant and enjoyed the pheasant immensely. To ensure that we made our plane back to Cleveland, we had to leave at 4:00 a.m. and drive the mountain route in the dark. That was a little scary but we arrived without mishap.

This morning we had breakfast at McDonald's in Calgary, turned in our car, and then caught our plane back to the states. We reversed the route on the return trip, flying into Houston before continuing on to Cleveland. At the Houston Airport there was a call for anyone who might be willing to relinquish their seats for the flight to Cleveland. Since we had left our car in Park 'N Fly we did not have to worry about anyone meeting us, so I turned in our names and waited to see what would happen. However, they did not need the seats so we returned to Cleveland on the regularly scheduled flight, picked up our car, and drove home.

Tuesday, January 26, 1999

We went to Dr. Koenig's office for a blood test and Muriel's WBC count of 2.9 was outside the lower range but not critical to her well-being. She saw Dr. Koenig briefly, as she thought she was getting a sinus infection. He provided her with a prescription for Levaquin. After the blood test, we went to the radiation therapy department of the hospital where Muriel had a consultation with Dr. Walsh, the radiation oncologist. I was not permitted to accompany her and stayed in the waiting room while she met with him. After Muriel returned from her consultation, we set up an appointment for her simulation for Friday the 29th. As we left the office Muriel shared what Dr. Walsh had said.

"He told me there may be long-term side effects with the radiation."

"Other than those they had told us about already?"

"Well, yes and no. He went into more detail, talking about the risk

47

of rib fracture, fibrosis, lung scarring, failure to control the disease," she stated matter-of-factly, then added with a smile, "Nothing we can't handle."

I smiled back, though a bit less confidently than she had. It is easy to reflect on such statements of risk after the fact. However, "failure to control the disease" is not something one dwells on at the time it is stated. The positive attitude of Muriel, which has also rubbed off on me, just said that we were going to beat this onerous beast known as cancer.

On our way to the parking deck we stopped off at the Ritzman Pharmacy located across the street from the hospital. Dr. Walsh had suggested that she get some RadiaCare Gel. Applying this aloe-based salve would help to keep Muriel's skin soft and prevent it from drying out from the radiation application. We left the pharmacy and drove to New Earth where Muriel replenished some of the herbals she is taking. Sue Wells was not working today so we were unable to get any further update on the first meeting of the support group.

Friday, January 29, 1999

Muriel had a 3:00 appointment in the radiation therapy department of Summa Health System for what was termed radiation simulation. She was taken into the radiation therapy room and an indelible mark was put on her skin that would enable the technician to focus the radiation at the same spot each time she was to have a treatment. It was all completed in a matter of five minutes and we were on our way back home. If one were cynical, one might conclude that the simulation just represented an opportunity for the hospital to make additional funds.

Saturday, January 30, 1999

The day was January 30, 1960, and we had gone to the Fireside Inn in Paramus, New Jersey for dinner. We were celebrating our first wedding anniversary and enjoyed Duckling Rosé with asparagus and wild rice with pecan pie for dessert. Tonight, 39 years later to the day, we celebrated our 40th anniversary. We had not made any plans except to enjoy our traditional anniversary dinner, that same meal we first enjoyed so long ago and many times since, eschewing going out to celebrate and just enjoying the meal at home. We also took the opportunity to read the card we had given each other for the past three years. We had discovered the card in a little shop in Fairfield Glade, Tennessee and were touched by the words which were so meaningful for us. The sentiment of the card follows.

Anniversary Thoughts of the Day Our Love Began
by Michele Savicki

Do you remember the day you and I first met,
when all time stood still and destiny took us both by the hand?

With you in my life, all the pieces of my world fall into place.
My heart is awakened, and the emptiness I once felt disappears.

You are my friend when I am alone
and my lover when our passions burn deep.
You are my teacher when I must learn
and my guide when I need to see which way to go.

You are my sunshine when clouds bring rain,
and my hope when I feel I can't go on.
In return, I give to you all that I can possibly be.
My reward comes every time I see you smile.

Today, let's look back on all that we have shared
and all we have made it through,
and let's look forward to all that is yet to come.
I love you now and forever.

Happy Anniversary

So we enjoyed our meal with a glass of rosé left over from the meal preparation, and reflected on the 40 years that God has given us and many of the events that have transpired in our life together. We talked about reaching our 50th anniversary and really celebrating. I cleaned up after dinner and we had coffee and pie in the family room. Later we watched one of our "feel good" movies, *Sense and Sensibility*, and enjoyed each other's company.

< 3 >
ROUND ONE OF RADIATION

Tuesday, February 2, 1999

Today is Groundhog Day, and according to Punxsutawney Phil we are to have six more weeks of winter. Now if you are a skier, that is good news. However, there were many people who were not happy to hear the news out of Pennsylvania.

We again are heading to the radiation therapy department of Summa Health System where Muriel is to receive her first radiation treatment. It is the first of 33 treatments and will be done daily, with the exception of the weekends, and will last until March 19th.

Much like the day Muriel had her simulation, her first real treatment is over in less than a minute. There is a short period for set up and then she is zapped. And much like the waiting room for chemotherapy where you see the same persons time and again, so too is the radiation waiting room. However, since there is a rigid schedule, there are not as many persons waiting. We initially met Joyce who was waiting for her husband Tony to complete his radiation. Muriel met Tony on the fly as he came out and she was going in. He was about halfway through his treatment cycle. While Muriel was having her treatment, a Vietnamese couple came in, the wife in line for treatment after Muriel. So we were a happy little band that passed each other every morning. Tony would eventually be replaced by a young man in his late twenties who had two children that he was caring for. He found it extremely difficult to meet this schedule, having to find a sitter for them while he tried to fit in the radiation, then get them squared away while he went to work. He also indicated that the radiation was sapping his strength and he was finding it increasingly difficult to go to work after radiation. However, he was resolved to get it done, his comment mirroring what Muriel has said: "You do what you have to do."

Keeping company with these folks going through radiation therapy gives me more opportunities to reflect on whether there is ever a "good" time to have cancer. If you have young children, and particularly if you are a single parent, it would seem to be a very difficult time to have cancer. Some time ago we had a young mother in her twenties who taught at Redeemer Christian School and had a child of eight. She died from cancer, leaving a husband and young daughter to cope with the loss of a spouse and mother. I had mentioned that Muriel and I had attended the funeral of one of the members of our church who was in her 60s when she passed away from cancer. It was of course a great loss to her husband and her family.

Can one say that now is a good time for Muriel to have cancer? Frankly, when thinking about all of the things one is subjected to when having cancer, never is obviously a good time to have cancer. That being said though, in a way I feel that we are fortunate that Muriel can at least face her cancer having had decades to develop a depth of faith and a broad life experience. Would she cope as well as she has was she in her twenties?

When faced with having cancer, I believe how one deals with it is of utmost importance. I am firmly convinced that Muriel's prayer for peace and God's granting of that peace has sustained her through all the facets of the treatment process. Because of her extraordinary attitude regarding this adventure of hers, I have a great sense that God will sustain us and all will be well.

Friday, February 5, 1999

The trips for radiation therapy have gotten routine. I drop Muriel off at the main entrance of the hospital, and she walks on through to the radiation therapy treatment center while I park the car. By the time I get to the center, she has removed her outer clothing and has slipped into a hospital gown. Then there is a short wait before she is called into the room for her treatment. In addition to radiation therapy, Muriel had a session with the radiation oncologist, Dr. Desiree Doncals. She had a wonderful manner and was very thorough in her examination of Muriel and in the explanations she provided. And unlike the other radiation oncologists, she welcomed my accompaniment of Muriel into the examination room. Since it is early in the radiation cycle Muriel is not yet affected by it.

We also went to Dr. Koenig's office to have a blood test. The WBC, RBC, and platelet counts were all in the acceptable ranges. On our way home we stopped at New Earth to pick up an additional supply of Greens & More. Sue Wells was working, so Muriel had a chance to talk with her and found out that the first meeting of the support group will be in March. After we got home, Muriel relaxed and I ran some errands. In the evening we went to the Outback Steakhouse for dinner, and then went to see a road company performance of the Broadway show *The King and I* at E. J. Thomas Hall.

Sunday, February 7, 1999

Today we went to church as usual but received the news that Bill Jenkins had died. Bill is the husband of Lois Jenkins, a member of the Chorale. Lois is also a Stephen Minister and had been assigned to Muriel to be her spiritual right arm as she moved forward on her adventure. Right after church we drove over to their house to see if we could lend comfort and solace to Lois. Though her son had not yet arrived, her three daughters and their families were already at her side. However, Lois was glad to see Muriel as they had grown quite close through her visits to see Muriel as her Stephen Minister. Bill suffered from emphysema and Lois had kept Muriel informed of his failing health during their times together. Nevertheless, when death actually comes it is a shock to those who are left behind, especially the spouse. We were there about two hours and departed when Pastor Johnson arrived.

Wednesday, February 10, 1999

We went to the funeral of Bill Jenkins today. Though I cherish life, as a Christian it is always heartwarming to know that an individual you count as a friend has gone to be with the Lord. One can also observe that this knowledge is comforting for those who are grieving the loss of a loved one. I don't know whether Muriel had a sense that maybe that would be me at some future point in time, but she held my hand a little tighter as we sat through the service. It was solemn, but with an uplifting message of life eternal for those who place their trust in the saving grace of Jesus Christ.

Friday, February 12, 1999

After radiation therapy this morning we returned home and I then proceeded to do my Friday exercises. I had open heart surgery in December of 1983 and continue to be an exercise buff, a routine I began in January 1977. I have a treadmill and a NordicTrack and I am on them six days a week, using Sunday as a recovery day. At the time I had my operation, Muriel switched us to a diet of chicken, fish, turkey, and vegetarian meals, and maybe red meat thrown in once or twice a month. This was all incorporated into the monthly meal schedule that Muriel prepared. It never ceases to amaze me what they can do with turkey. We have had turkey ham, turkey sausage, turkey breakfast sausage, turkey Italian sausage, turkey kielbasa, and turkey pepperoni. All of those delicious foods could still be eaten if prepared in a more health-conscious way, and Muriel took full advantage of that fact, offering diverse choices we both enjoyed. In short, she took care of us, of me, and I tried my best to do the same for her.

Tonight though, we were eating out. In the evening we headed to Cleveland for a Cleveland Orchestra concert and stopped at Charley's Crab House just off of I-271 on Chagrin Boulevard. We each had a green salad with a house dressing that was just great. I had the blackened mahi-mahi and Muriel settled for a grilled tuna steak. We both enjoyed the meal and continue to give thanks to the Lord for the blessings He gives us daily.

We don't do it each time we dine out, but tonight we both reflected on the journey Muriel had made in her life, at one point touching upon a turning point in our lives over two decades ago. Muriel and I had gone on a Marriage Encounter weekend after we had been married 18 years. Prior to that time Muriel's self-image was quite negative. She could do 99 things right and one thing wrong, and she would dwell on the one thing she had done wrong. I on the other hand could do 99 things wrong and one thing right and I would dwell on the one thing right. Her saying about me was *Hand Keith a lemon and he will make lemonade.* For me the glass was always half full, and for her it was always half empty.

The Marriage Encounter weekend was the impetus for Muriel to make a dramatic change in her life. She came to the realization that self-image meant exactly that, how you view yourself. She was always a perfectionist because her parents seemed, in my view, to always expect her to be the best, and if she were not it was a case of *Why not?* That is a ton of pressure. She graduated summa cum laude from undergraduate school, and had nothing but A's as she earned an M.A. at the University of Akron, yet she was still so hard on herself. Her parents were both alcoholics and she carried the gene as well, often seeking solace in alcohol. But now all of that is behind her and she so likes herself that it enables her to reach out and embrace others, and tell them what the Lord has done in her life. At the culmination of our conversation she said something that affirmed what I had contemplated might be true, regarding my thoughts on a "good" time to have cancer.

"If I had had cancer back then I wouldn't have been able to handle it. I probably would have died shortly after the diagnosis."

"Perhaps," I said, "but I guess we'll never know for sure. One thing is certain though."

"What's that?"

"You are stronger now than you have ever been since we met," I answered. "Strong in every way the word can measure."

She saw my eyes water a bit and smiled. I returned the gesture and we both laughed a bit at the comforting thought. Can you imagine going through what she is experiencing, and having a smile on her face and nothing but joy in her heart? I truly meant what I had said. Muriel was stronger than ever in my opinion, and I was sure that her strength had made me stronger as well. Our dinner was delicious, but we were especially delighted in the reflection of the past and thoughts of our future, leaving the restaurant hand in hand and with spirits high.

We went straight from one high to the next as the Cleveland Orchestra, under the direction of Jahja Ling, began the program with one of our all time favorites, *Adagio for Strings* by Samuel Barber. It is a piece that many may remember from the movie *The Apocalypse.* The Cleveland Orchestra played the piece so beautifully. Joshua Bell was the soloist on the second piece, entitled *The Red Violin: Chaconne* by John Corigliano. The last presentation before intermission was *Three Pieces from Schindler's List* by John Williams. After intermission the orchestra was joined by the Cleveland Orchestra Chorus for Sergei Prokofiev's *Alexander Nevsky.* Even though the long, full day had grown late and cold, we were two happy campers on our ride back home to Munroe Falls.

Monday, February 15, 1999

After radiation therapy today, Muriel spent some time with Dr. Demas, one of the interchangeable radiation oncologists. "It is great to see that you are tolerating the treatment very well," he said. "Even your skin is showing just mild radiation changes."

"Thanks to Keith," Muriel said. My applications of the RadiaCare Gel were doing a good job of keeping Muriel's skin supple and not letting it dry out. Every night before Muriel went to bed I would spend time rubbing the area of the back where the radiation was given. The exact location was not difficult to find since there was an indelible mark which pinpointed the area to be covered. I was happy to hear that my efforts were of some help.

Wednesday, February 17, 1999

Today is Ash Wednesday and a long standing tradition at our church is to have congregational dinners during Lent. I think it was done to accommodate working families as well as offer an enticement to come to the Lenten service. Tonight's meal was chicken with mashed potatoes, green beans, salad, and rolls. That portion of the meal was catered, but the desserts were supplied by the parishioners unless they chose to have ice cream. Tonight they had several pies from which to choose. A basket at the beginning of the line allowed those who participated to make a free-will offering to help defray the expense. Muriel and I were among the first to be fed because the Chorale was singing and we had to rehearse prior to the service. The Chorale had prepared four numbers. We experienced the imposition of ashes and also partook of the Lord's Supper. Muriel got many "atta-girls" both before and after the service which just added to her positive self-image. At this stage she has lost all of her hair and just proceeds to wear hats as a protection against the cold. She no longer gets any comments about being bald.

Thursday, February 18, 1999

In addition to radiation therapy, today we stopped in Dr. Koenig's office so Muriel could have a blood test. With the exception of the RBC count the WBCs and platelets were within the acceptable range. I continue to marvel at Muriel's stamina and resilience as she continues with radiation therapy with no apparent side effects to her well-being. For all of the blood tests she has had, at no time has she been told that there is a problem and she would not be able to have chemotherapy or radiation. In my judgment, Muriel's positive mental attitude that *God is in charge* serves her well in all of the therapies she has had. It has also been so very uplifting to me and to all those whom she meets.

Friday, February 19, 1999

It was good to get back home after radiation therapy, inside and away from the blustery weather outside. I lit a fire in the fireplace and we pretty much cooled it for the day. I did venture out to take some of the accumulated magazines to the recycle place and to put gas in the car. At 5:00 we headed for Cleveland. We stopped at the China Gate Restaurant where Muriel had Orange Beef and I had Kung Po Chicken. Since we could leave food in the car without fear of spoilage, Muriel got a "doggie bag" for the remainder of her meal. I have become pretty adept at eating with chopsticks; in fact, our waiter was convinced that I was a native of the San Francisco area because of my technique. However, I had to disabuse him of that idea.

After dinner we continued down Cedar Road heading to Severance Hall where we heard the Cleveland Orchestra, under the direction of Oliver Knussen, play Stravinsky's *Scenes de Ballet*, followed by two pieces by Toru Takemitsu, *Riverrun* and *Asterism*. After intermission, Peter Serkin was the piano soloist on a piece by Alexander Scriabin entitled *The Poem of Ecstasy*. Not only was it a late night driving back to Munroe Falls, but it was a cold night as well.

Monday, February 22, 1999

"Happy anniversary," I said to Muriel as she walked into the kitchen for breakfast.

"Happy anniversary, sweetie," she replied, pecking me on the cheek. It was not like the anniversary of our marriage, but it was always a date that we acknowledged to each other. It was the day that we first met in 1958.

I was a freshman at Clarkson College of Technology in Potsdam, New York. Muriel's sister, Judith, was a freshman at the State University of New York at Potsdam. Judith and I had met because I had a car and would transport her and other students to Massena, New York to go to the Lutheran Church, the closest one to Potsdam. Judith and I had also had several social outings because we liked to dance. Muriel had just broken an engagement and her mother suggested that she travel to Potsdam to visit her sister. She took the train from Grand Central Station in New York City to Potsdam, a trip that took a day and a half, and it wasn't even a sleeper.

It was Ice Carnival weekend and since I was a veteran, Judith chose me to escort her sister for the weekend. Judith lived in the Elm Street dorm, a Quonset hut that housed 24 students. I had been asked to come to the dorm on Friday afternoon to meet Muriel before our scheduled date in the evening.

As the story is told after the fact, I apparently did not make a very good impression at this introductory meeting. There was a single chair in the vestibule where I had set myself down to await Muriel's entry. When Muriel came into the vestibule I did not rise to offer her the seat and thus received a black mark. It was almost a deal-breaker because Muriel told her sister that she wanted out of the evening date. However, Judith went to bat for me and convinced Muriel that she should go on the date and try and make the most of it.

We went to a hockey game between Clarkson and Colgate. Muriel did not know much about hockey, so I had the opportunity to redeem myself a bit by explaining all of the nuances of the game to her as the periods unfolded. After the game, which Clarkson won, we went to a Vets Club party that was held at Green's, a college hangout, in Hannawa Falls. We had a few beers, danced to records on the jukebox and talked and talked. Since the girls in the dorm had curfews back then, I had to have Muriel back by 1:00. I walked her to the door, gave her a big hug and kissed her good night. I climbed into my car thinking that maybe I had found the love of my life. She told me sometime later that she fell in love with me that night. We were married 11 months later on January 30, 1959.

After breakfast Muriel went to have her radiation therapy and met again with Dr. Demas, the radiation oncologist on duty this morning, for a progress report. "So far, so good Muriel. You are doing remarkably well," he said, "so we'll continue the treatment course as we planned." We were both obviously glad to hear this, and I again offered God a prayer of thanks.

Right after our meeting, Muriel waited at the hospital while I went across the street to Ritzman Pharmacy to get another tube of RadiaCare Gel. I then picked her up and we drove to New Earth to get some additional herbals that she needed. Sue Wells was at the store and offered Muriel more details about the first support group meeting. It would be held the first Saturday in March in the back room of Treasures From Heaven, a keepsake store on Bailey Road in Cuyahoga Falls. Sue wasn't exactly sure how many people would be there, but she had invited eight women to attend. We thanked Sue and left, but I realized Muriel hadn't told Sue whether or not she would be attending the first meeting.

"Do you think you'll go?" Judging by her excitement, I was sure I knew the answer.

"To the meeting? I wouldn't miss it. I'm really looking forward to sharing our experiences with each other. It'll be great. It's one thing to share a bit of my adventure with some folks going through a similar experience in a waiting room. It's another thing entirely to gather specifically to share our experiences, to share our knowledge, our hope, our laughter. I can't wait."

I hadn't seen Muriel so excited in quite some time, and it was infectious. We went home and continued our conversation as we enjoyed lunch. Afterward Muriel made a bowl of popcorn and climbed into her waterbed to read and relax while I went to Boston Mills to take my skis in for waxing and edging. The entire time I was out, I thought about Muriel's adventure and realized finally what the support group means to her. She hadn't even attended a meeting, yet the group has already impacted her and lifted her spirits. I knew Muriel would get so much from her support group, but I also realized that her story was an important one to share with them as well. As she had inspired many who knew her, perhaps she could now inspire many more who were on their own adventures with cancer. I am excited for her, and the elevated mood continued into the evening as Muriel faithfully and energetically directed the Chorale practice.

Friday, February 26, 1999

In addition to the radiation therapy we stopped off in Dr. Koenig's office so Muriel could have her port flushed and have a blood test. We sat for a short saline drip at which time blood was drawn. The WBC count and the platelets were within the acceptable range. The RBC count was below the acceptable range but apparently did not set off any alarms. All of these therapies and tests had become so routine for us that it became *just another day at the office*. We were soon on our way back home.

"When we get home, I'm going to curl up in my La-Z-Boy with one of my books," she said, "and I think you should go skiing."

"Well I hadn't planned on it and—"

"And you hadn't planned on spending all of your time carting me around either. You deserve a little break, no?"

I started to protest but she insisted I take some time to enjoy myself. So while she relaxed at home I went to Boston Mills to ski. Please realize that Ohio does not have any mountains and not even many very steep hills, but there are places to ski and Boston Mills is one of them, together with its sister location Brandywine. At both places it is about four-and-a-half minutes to the top by lift and only 30 seconds back down to the bottom of the hill. However, Boston Mills has been great for me and has allowed me to develop my parallel skiing technique. I was very thankful for Muriel's suggestion to ski as I skied for about four hours. I enjoyed myself immensely and kept thinking I'd do one more run and then go, only to make another, and another. I was back home by 3:00 and Muriel was preparing herself for our evening date, dinner at Mario's Eastside Restaurant followed with a performance by Ohio Ballet. Ohio Ballet gives three performances in their subscription series and this was the penultimate.

Monday, March 1, 1999

On Mondays during radiation therapy there is always a visit with the radiation oncologist. Today we met with Dr. Doncals before she had therapy. The examination included checking vital signs and then some pressure exercises to see if Muriel had lost any strength.

Muriel told Dr. Doncals she was mostly doing well. "I have been experiencing shortness of breath lately, especially yesterday, but it's fine today."

She asked Muriel some questions and offered her recommendations. "We'll have you get a chest X-ray and MUGA scan and then compare them to the earlier ones to see if we can figure out why that's happening," Dr. Doncals said. "Overall, though, you seem to be doing great. I see no reason to change our treatment plans."

While Muriel was in for her radiation therapy, I made arrangements for a MUGA scan which she would have on Wednesday. From radiation therapy we stopped at the outpatient laboratory for a chest X-ray and then went home to relax for the day.

Wednesday, March 3, 1999

Today we began with a trip to radiation therapy and then we stayed at the hospital where Muriel had a MUGA scan. We will have to wait for our next visit with Dr. Doncals to find out the results.

Friday, March 5, 1999

This morning we followed the regular routine for radiation therapy session number 23. I drop Muriel off at the entrance to the hospital. I park the car. She walks through the hospital to the radiation therapy department and changes into a hospital gown, and returns to sit with me until she is called in for her treatment. We both could probably do it blindfolded at this time. That is said not to indicate that it is boring, but because it is such a practiced routine, a routine she has shown up for every day. It seems they all do. Those who have not experienced cancer have little idea what patients go through to overcome the disease. Thank God that the human spirit is so remarkably resilient.

After radiation therapy we took the elevator to the second floor in the hospital, crossed the bridge between the hospital and the physician's office building, and went to Dr. Koenig's office so Muriel could have a blood test. Getting a blood test in Dr. Koenig's office provides immediate feedback, as the technician has a machine that analyzes the blood draw seconds after it is taken. Thus, we knew before we left the office that the WBC count was just slightly below the acceptable level and that the RBC count and platelets were satisfactory. As before, she can still continue to have radiation.

Saturday, March 6, 1999

While I got out the vacuum and cleaned the living room and dining room, Muriel was off to her first support group meeting. She returned a little after 3:00 and was very eager to share her experience. "For starters, I'm the oldest," she said.

"Of how many?"

"There were six others besides me. Sue of course, and Robin Graham who we both met. Then there was Linda Allen, Carol Wheeler, Jan Margida, and Nancy Libengood. We each shared our personal story and discussed what stage of treatment each of us is in and just talked about it, about life with it, life before it. About our futures. It was a wonderful experience."

"Sounds like it."

"We laughed together, we cried together. I could really feel the support from each one of them. By the way, I was put in charge of laughter."

"What does that mean?"

"It means that each time we meet I have to bring something that will give us a good laugh."

We had a good laugh at that and continued to talk about the meeting for a long while, perhaps longer than the meeting itself. I could almost cut Muriel's eagerness with a knife as she, for the first time, worked on making the group laugh. We both looked forward to her next meeting.

Monday, March 8, 1999

Today was "meet with the radiation oncologist" day and since Dr. Heater was the oncologist of record, I was not able to accompany Muriel into the session. When we were reunited, I asked, "What did Dr. Heater have to say?"

"Just the same as Dr. Doncals said last week, that I was doing great."

Afterward Muriel again suggested that I go skiing. She knows how much I enjoy skiing and is trying hard to make our lives as normal as possible. So I suited up and went to Boston Mills. I skied until about 3:30 when busloads of schoolkids began to arrive and the slopes got crowded and dangerous. I stopped at Acme on the way home and picked up a loaf of French bread, arriving home in time to make dinner. It was easy—we were having spaghetti with turkey Italian sausage. I sliced the French bread open, added butter and garlic salt, and then wrapped it up in aluminum foil and put it in the oven. To accent that, we added a little glass of rosé and had a delightful dinner together. These are the times spent together, watching the news as we have our dinner and just doing the things we normally do, that make the happenings in our lives seem so unreal. God really has given us peace of mind, and further, it seems He never sends us more than we can bear.

Tuesday, March 9, 1999

After dropping Muriel off at the hospital I stopped over at Ritzman's Pharmacy and picked up another tube of RadiaCare Gel. We have been very attentive to using it every evening, particularly at the point of the radiation therapy, and Muriel continues to get good marks for skin care. Muriel was already in getting her therapy by the time I arrived. I got my parking pass validated, which meant I didn't have to pay for parking. This was just another part of the routine. Although the expense of the parking would not have been prohibitive, it was a nice gesture on the part of Summa Health System to include the cost of parking as part of the radiation therapy service.

The completion of the radiation therapy coincided with our scheduled Stephen Leaders meeting. We drove to Cuyahoga Falls and Redeemer Lutheran Church where we met in Pastor Larry's office and mapped out training exercises, Stephen Ministry assignments, and future activities. After dinner we were right back at church where Muriel directed the practice of the Chorale. Considering she is always in a hat these days, many people are always on the lookout to see if it is a new one, or at least a style different from the one she was wearing the last time they saw her. She does not disappoint. She has ordered another six hats from Eddie Bauer to add to her expanding collection.

Wednesday, March 10, 1999

After the early session of radiation therapy we returned home and I did my usual Wednesday exercises consisting of the treadmill,

NordicTrack, sit-ups, push-ups, and other stretches. That accomplished, I showered and ran several errands, including going to the bank, getting gas for the car, going to Penney's, stopping at the card shop, and finally, stopping in to see Anna Klippel. Anna is the oldest person in our congregation and she is not feeling well. She has been married for 63 years and is just a delight with whom to visit. After conversing with her I ultimately said a prayer for her recovery and departed.

Muriel and I went to the Lenten dinner at church and then to the Lenten service. The Chorale sang two numbers and Muriel received plaudits from members of the congregation as we left for home. She so enjoys being the director and seems to pick out just the right music to complement the voices she has available to sing.

Friday, March 12, 1999

Radiation therapy session number 28. Once again it was the normal routine: drop Muriel off at the door, then park the car while she walks through the hospital to the therapy room and changes into a hospital gown. By then I have gotten my parking ticket stamped and she is about to be called in for her radiation. Everything is so efficient. After therapy we continue up to Dr. Koenig's office where she has her blood drawn. All counts are in the acceptable ranges so radiation continues.

Saturday, March 13, 1999

Muriel slept until nearly 1:00 today and then proceeded to lounge in the family room. I added to the ambience of the room by lighting a fire in our fireplace. There seemed to be a slight chill but soon the warmth from the fire permeated every corner of the room. It was another of those special times, quietly enjoying each other's company and feeling truly blessed, the warmth sustaining us until it was time to get ready to go out.

We went to dinner at a brewery pub in Merriman Valley right near the Weathervane Playhouse. They had a sampler of three of the beers they brew so we tested all three and then ordered the "lively lager." We began the meal with a garden fresh salad. I cast the cholesterol thing aside for tonight and ordered a steak medium rare, a baked potato with sour cream, and the grilled veggies. Muriel had a shrimp dish, rice pilaf, and the grilled veggies as well. The food was excellent.

After we ate we drove a short distance to the Weathervane Playhouse where we had tickets for the performance of *Madame Butterfly*. All of the music was very good but the soprano aria "Un bel di" was just exquisite. The story is very touching and we held hands while it unfolded.

Monday, March 15, 1999

Today marked visit number 29 for radiation therapy and it was also Monday, so that meant a visit with the radiation oncologist. Dr. Doncals was on duty today so I got to accompany Muriel into the examination room. The bedside manner of Dr. Doncals is outstanding, and each time we see her it is like visiting with a close friend or relative. She was very thorough in her questioning and in her hands-on examination. She said, "Both the X-ray and the MUGA scan were negative, so hopefully whatever it was that was causing your shortness of breath has passed. You'll be seeing your other doctors in the coming weeks and we'll see you back here in one month."

"Thank you for taking care of Muriel," I said, reaching to shake her hand.

"You're welcome. It has been my pleasure. Oh, and keep up your part with the RadiaCare Gel. You can see the difference it makes."

"I promise I will and I will keep to it."

Friday, March 19, 1999

Six weeks plus three days and we finally arrive at the 33rd and last radiation therapy treatment. The day was no different than all the previous sessions. Drop Muriel off at the entrance to the hospital. I then park the car while she walks to the radiation therapy department and changes. I bring my parking ticket to the desk to get it stamped and then move to the radiation therapy waiting room to hold Muriel's purse while she gets her treatment. We drove back home when the session was completed and contemplated the next course of action. She will have a few days off and then begin the next round of chemotherapy.

During the period of time Muriel experienced radiation therapy her hair has started to grow back. She is still wearing one of her hats each time she goes out, but she has a good start with a one-and-a-half inch growth. Alas, it is all to fall out again with the next round of chemotherapy.

In the meantime, our lives are back to normal, or as normal as can be with further chemotherapy in the future. It is now almost six months since Muriel's adventure began, and nearly eight months will have passed before all of the treatments are completed. We were informed of all of the things that would take place throughout Muriel's treatment the very first time we met with Dr. Koenig and spoke with one of his oncology nurses. However, at that time it seemed a little overwhelming. As previously noted, I suspect that not many people, outside of family and friends, realize what a cancer patient goes through in the process of his or her treatment. Now that I have witnessed the tremendous efforts firsthand, I will never think of cancer or those diagnosed with it the same way again.

We now settled into our regular routines. I am up early and do my exercises and Muriel sleeps in until 10:00 or 11:00, or perhaps even later. I run errands or work on a jigsaw puzzle which is spread out on the dining room table. Muriel has been doing most of the cooking and we eat in the family room using TV tables while we watch "Live on Five," and then the local and national news on ABC.

Usually on Sundays, Muriel peruses the television schedule of the *Akron Beacon Journal* and determines what she plans on watching on television for the week. I of course am happy to watch any sporting event that is being broadcast. Since we still have only one television (I know you are thinking *Only one television?*), unless the sporting event has the New York Rangers, New York Giants, or especially the New York Yankees, I am happy to give up the set to see the program Muriel has chosen.

We often watch *Mystery* on PBS, *Biography* on A&E, or *Inside the Actors Studio* on Bravo. We also watch other programs on PBS as well as those on the History Channel. Network television is just not viewed in our house with the exception of news and investigative programs such as *60 Minutes* or *20/20*, or other specials that appeal to us. If there is nothing of interest we often choose to view one of the 600 videos that we have accumulated through Muriel's purchases and recordings. And of course, reading is always a ready alternative. With 3,000 volumes in the house there is never a problem in finding something to read.

Friday, March 26, 1999

We often go out to dinner on the nights that we have tickets to the Akron Symphony Orchestra, but tonight's dinner also served as a celebration of the completion of the radiation therapy portion of Muriel's treatment. We decided to do something different, so we went to the Japanese restaurant in the Merriman Valley and sat at a table for eight where the cook prepared all of the food right in front of us. He surely knew how to wield his knife and spatula, performing flips with his utensils as he prepared and served all of the different ingredients of our meal. It was an excellent, entertaining meal and, even though we shared it with others, just being together enjoying ourselves was truly satisfying.

After dinner we went to E. J. Thomas Hall where we enjoyed the Akron Symphony Orchestra. The conductor for the evening was David Wiley and he had selected a unique program. All three pieces were entitled *Romeo and Juliet* by three separate composers beginning with Berlioz, then Prokofiev, and lastly Tchaikovsky. It was an interesting evening as we listened to the way each of the composers dealt with Shakespeare's star-crossed lovers. We are very familiar with the Tchaikovsky version and enjoyed that one the most.

Thursday, April 1, 1999

Muriel had an appointment today with Dr. Koenig regarding the new round of chemotherapy. We had not been to his office in some time but it was still jam-packed with patients waiting to see the doctor or to have treatment. Although Muriel continues to be at peace with her adventure, for me, seeing all of these persons in various stages of dealing with their cancer is difficult. How many would survive? How many would fully recover? Would Muriel survive? Would she fully recover? How many lives had been affected by the onset of cancer? We were all just grains of sand in the desert of life.

I was brought back to reality when nurse Pattie called on us. Initially Muriel had a blood test, and the WBC and RBC counts were in the acceptable range. The platelets were slightly elevated but the high side was not critical. Next she was weighed (122 pounds) and moved into an examination room where the nurse took her blood pressure (130/80) and brought her file up to date. Muriel provided her with a new list of all of the meds she is presently taking. Dr. Koenig arrived soon after and began a discussion of the benefits and risks of the Taxol treatment.

"Taxol interferes with the growth of cancer cells and slows their spread in the body, but it can lower your white blood cell count, and the white blood cells are what help your body to fight infection. In light of this, are you still willing to continue the treatment?"

Without hesitation and with a quick glance at me she answered, "Of course, let's continue."

He said, "All right. It's even more important that we have your blood tested regularly as you have the Taxol treatment and we'll keep a close eye on all of your counts. We'll see you next Thursday."

It seemed fitting that we heard all about the next round of chemotherapy on April Fools' Day. We departed and the unanswered questions that had crossed my mind in the waiting room made their return.

< 4 >
CHEMOTHERAPY: ROUND TWO

Friday, April 2, 1999

Today was a routine Friday. Muriel slept in and I was up early and did my usual exercises. I ran several errands, one of which was to have a prescription filled for dexamethasone that Dr. Koenig had provided in anticipation of Muriel's next round of chemotherapy. In the afternoon I caught up on the paperwork associated with my job as secretary of the Stow Senior Men's Golf League that plays on Wednesday mornings at the Fox Den Golf Course in Stow. At 5:30 we drove to Cleveland for a concert at Severance Hall. We stopped at the China Gate Restaurant where we each again ordered our favorite Chinese dinner: Muriel had the Orange Beef with vegetables and I had Kung Po Chicken. We both had white rice and shared a pot of Chinese tea. As we began eating, Muriel revived the conversation we had on our way back from Texas. "Do you think I should have a prophylactic removal of my left breast?"

I responded in much the same way I had before, though this time without delay. "It's not my decision to make."

"No, I know it isn't, but I know you can help me to decide."

She smiled at me and I of course melted. I really did feel like a fish out of water but wanted to help her the best I could to make the choice that was best for her. Muriel continued, rehashing her argument in favor of a second mastectomy.

"If the breast isn't there then the chances of getting breast cancer again do not exist."

"You don't need to convince me."

"I know, but I just want to know how you feel about it."

"You know how I feel, sweetie. I'll do whatever you need me to do and I will support you in any decision you make that you feel is right for you." She blushed a bit and I continued, proffering the same suggestion I had made before. "I do think it is important to speak with your doctors. Their opinions matter far more than my own. Would you be ready for another operation after this next round of chemo, for instance? I don't know, but they would."

"You're right, I'll talk to them," she said, looking at her hands and then up at me again. "I do think I should have the breast removed and eliminate some of the risk of the cancer returning."

"Then that's what we'll do and we'll talk to the doctors about making that happen," I said, relaxing a bit. "If they're on board, we'll have them write letters of recommendation since I'm sure our insurance will require it. And then you'll have the operation and we'll see where the adventure takes us from there."

With that she smiled again, but some of my anxiety remained. There is no question in my mind that when the second round of chemotherapy is complete the adventure will continue. Where it will take us I have no idea. I guess that accounted for most of the anxiety. But any doubts I may have had were put to rest at least temporarily when she said, "I think I'll have the port removed at the same time too."

"Why not?" I concurred. I had faith God was removing all the cancer from her body with her treatment, so why would she need a port? We enjoyed our dinner and then made our way to Severance Hall. The Cleveland Orchestra opened their program with a world premiere piece entitled *Cantigas* by Magnus Lindberg and the second half of the program featured *The Song of the Earth* by Gustav Mahler. The latter was a choral piece featuring the orchestra and solo voices. It was a usual ponderous piece by Mahler, but enjoyable. As we got into spring, the drive home from Cleveland was less tedious but nonetheless it was another late night.

Thursday, April 8, 1999

Today it started all over again. At 8:30 we departed for Dr. Koenig's office for the second round of chemotherapy. The waiting room was near capacity with individuals waiting to see the doctor or to receive treatment. Wives accompanied husbands. Husbands attended their wives. Daughters helped with mothers. Sons or daughters kept dads company. And some just braved the ordeal all alone.

If Muriel ever felt depressed at the sight of all of these persons traveling the cancer road, and she has a history of depression, she never once seemed to be affected. I hung up our jackets and she reported to the front desk to let them know she was here for her chemotherapy. She was soon called and we returned to the chemotherapy room, the same chair in the corner, in fact, for the first infusion of Taxol.

Since it had been nearly four months since the initial chemotherapy, there was a complete turnover in the individuals who occupied the other chairs in the room. The new group of patients in the room was more subdued than the previous individuals, so there was little exchange between the patients as each sat and waited for the incessant drip of the fluids to be complete.

Needless to say, Muriel is extremely happy that she had a port put in place. All of the blood tests she has had, and now more chemotherapy, are much easier with a port. Prior to our departure from home, she had put a little EMLA cream on the skin over the port area. Then there is little or no pain when the needle is inserted.

The three nurses, working with individual patients, are very efficient in setting up each IV bag and getting the patient comfortable. Initially the nurse caring for Muriel introduced medications into her IV line (Zofran, Zantac, and Benadryl) that would help to relieve nausea and the discomfort of the chemotherapy. Each medication had a prescribed drip time and after they all entered into her system, the bag containing the Taxol was introduced. The drip time for that was approximately one hour.

Both Muriel and I had brought something to read, so I sat on the stool at her feet and read, stroking her arm occasionally. After the hour had passed she received a saline flush and we were on our way home. Although she wasn't nauseous, Muriel was reluctant to have anything for lunch, so I had an eight-ounce container of yogurt and then, with her blessing, I went to play bridge at church.

Wednesday, April 14, 1999

Muriel had a 3:00 appointment with Dr. Walsh, one of the radiation oncologists she had seen during the radiation therapy. It was her one-month follow-up and I sat in the waiting room while she met with him. When she returned I asked, "How did it go?"

"Fine. He said my skin looks good and we'll follow-up again in a month."

"Did you ask him what he thought about having your other breast removed?"

"Yes, he agreed it's a good idea, and he also agreed to write a letter of recommendation for me."

"That sounds good."

"I guess we'll see what Dr. Flynn has to say about it tomorrow and go from there." We made our way home with Muriel in high spirits. I am happy for her, but at the same time a bit somber about the prospects of her having to undergo another operation.

Thursday, April 15, 1999

This morning Muriel had an appointment in Dr. Koenig's office to have a blood test. Just as was necessary with the first round of chemotherapy, it is important to keep track of the red blood cells, white blood cells, and platelets. It is necessary to avoid neutropenia, which occurs when white blood cell counts are very low, or thrombocytopenia, which occurs when platelet counts are very low. Should either of those deficiencies occur, it would be necessary to stop the chemotherapy until such time as the deficiencies were rectified. Thus, between the delivery of the chemotherapy drug sessions, it is necessary to have weekly blood tests. The RBC count was 4.14, the WBC count was 2.4, and the platelet count was 270. The WBC count was below the acceptable range but apparently did not set off any signals as to it being critical. There were still several weeks before Muriel will have another round of chemotherapy.

After the blood test we took the elevator to the 4th floor where Muriel had an appointment with Dr. Flynn. Her main purpose was to broach the subject of having her other breast removed, and at the same time have the port taken out. Dr. Flynn also supported the idea of having her left breast removed, and he too indicated that he would be willing to write a letter attesting to the need for such a procedure. Tentative plans were made for the procedure, but nothing would be done until she had finished her second round of chemotherapy. On the way to the parking deck I said, "Well, that's two down and two to go." Muriel just gave me a big smile.

Friday, April 16, 1999

We continue to move forward with our lives and have settled into the routine of chemotherapy followed by periodic blood tests, as contrasted to the daily trip to receive the radiation therapy. Muriel pretty much continues to be in charge of our home life and all of the activities that are encompassed in that statement. I have certain routines which are my domain, such as cleaning up after every meal, doing the dishes, making the beds, and fetching and toting things around the house as the need arises. I am also a great errand runner.

This evening Muriel and I went out to dinner and then on to the Ohio Ballet presentation in the Akron Civic Theatre. Since the theater is located on Main Street in downtown Akron, we were home just 15 minutes after the program was complete.

Thursday, April 22, 1999

This morning Muriel had an appointment for a blood test in Dr. Koenig's office. The WBC count was below the acceptable range, but the RBC count and platelets were in the acceptable range, so apparently we are still a go for the next session of chemotherapy.

Inadvertently I just typed "we" rather than "Muriel" or "she." As time progresses it becomes more apparent to me that even though I am not getting the chemotherapy, I am not getting the blood tests, and I am not taking the CT scans and X-rays, I am still an integral part of the activity that surrounds all of those undertakings.

From the medical center we went to New Earth to pick up more herbal supplements. Sue Wells was not working today so we picked up the items that were needed and continued on home.

Friday, April 23, 1999

The day was noteworthy because I got out the clippers and, using a number two rake, I cut off Muriel's hair again. The hair had returned after the first session of chemotherapy but was somewhat spotty and seemed to be at varying lengths. Since her hair was all due to fall out as a result of the Taxol, Muriel wanted to have it all the same length. She had been wearing hats all through the radiation therapy and right up to the present. However, even though it wasn't long she did not want it to be "messy" as she put it.

In the evening we drove to the Outback Steakhouse in Macedonia, a stopover on our way to another Cleveland Orchestra concert. Muriel had the petite steak and I had "Ribs on the Barbie." I relished my ribs with a Foster's draft. As we are into daylight savings time, the drive to Cleveland was in the daylight. We enjoyed the scenery as the trees were beginning to bud and here and there crocuses were displaying their spring colors. The Cleveland Orchestra featured Pierre Boulez as the guest conductor who began the evening with Maurice Ravel's

Pavane pour une infante défunte. It is an absolutely gorgeous piece and established a mood of warmth and closeness for the evening that grew as additional pieces were brought to the ears of the audience. The next three pieces were all composed by Claude Debussy and were entitled *Ballades de François Villon, Le jet d'eau,* and *Danses sacrée et profane.* The second half of the program was an opera in concert by Ravel entitled *L'enfant et les sortilèges.* There were five solo voices and the Cleveland Orchestra Chorus. It was the first time we had seen and heard an opera in concert, and it was very well done.

The drive back to Munroe Falls did not seem as long as it usually did in the winter months. It is amazing what effect the change in weather can have on one's whole outlook on life, and having been warmed and drawn closer by the music we shared, we zipped home in short order.

Wednesday, April 28, 1999

We met with Dr. Koenig to determine if Muriel could continue with the Taxol chemotherapy. When she was called into the office she was weighed (125 pounds) and had her blood pressure measured (138/84). After quizzing and examining Muriel, Dr. Koenig cleared her to continue the second round of chemotherapy. Before we left, Muriel said, "I'm thinking of having my left breast removed when I finish the Taxol treatments. Do you think that's a good idea?"

"If you don't have the breast, then I would guess you won't get breast cancer again."

"Exactly. Would you be willing to write a letter for my insurance company?"

"Absolutely. When do you need it?"

"I'll let you know."

When we left Dr. Koenig's office I told Muriel, "You just need a letter from Dr. Waugh."

"I'm sure he'll agree also."

I made a side trip to Ritzman's Pharmacy to pick up small glassine bags that we needed to carry pills for our next overseas trip. We then went directly home and began the preparation for our trip we had scheduled in the middle of Muriel's first round of chemotherapy.

Thursday, April 29, 1999

This morning we return to Dr. Koenig's office for the second round of Taxol infiltration. I think my car could find its own way to the parking deck at 92 Arch Street if I would let it. It has been just three weeks since the initial session. Muriel had one of the seats in the row of chairs with the window at their backs. These chairs are a little closer together and I had to wait to sit by Muriel until the nurse got her IV hooked up. She started with the three medications to prevent nausea, and then came the large bag containing the Taxol. Time elapsed very quickly as we both had brought something to read. When her session ended I tried to keep the mood light and said, "Time sure flies when you're having fun." She had no comment but she did offer me a big grin. We returned home and continued our preparation to go overseas.

Sunday, May 2, 1999

Today we depart for an Elderhostel trip to Scandinavia. We are scheduled to spend five days in Copenhagen, Denmark, five days in Oslo, Norway, and five days in Stockholm, Sweden, plus a travel day. We left home in a state of excited anticipation.

Tuesday, May 18, 1999

We returned from our overseas journey last night, a little tired but renewed. The trip was all we had hoped for. We had one individual who served as the "mother hen" for the group and was responsible for getting us to the right place at the right time. In each city we would have a class in the morning in which a local guide would share about the architecture, economy, population, government, educational system, and other subjects deemed to be of interest to us.

Then, after lunch, we would take walking tours or bus tours in the area enjoying those things that tourists generally came to see. Thus in Copenhagen we saw the statue of the Little Mermaid and the home of Hans Christian Anderson, the outdoor market Strøget, and visited Tivoli. In Stockholm we saw the old city and visited Skansen, an open-air museum that depicts the early life of the Swedes. In Oslo, we visited the Viking Ship Museum, the ships of Thor Heyerdahl, the Vigeland Monolith, the Edvard Munch Museum and the famous Holmenkollen ski jump. Of course there were many other places to go and see and it was just a great 16 days.

One free afternoon when we were in Copenhagen, Muriel and I and another couple agreed to take a train ride to visit *Hamlet's* Kronborg Castle in Helsingør. We bought our train tickets, got ourselves on the right platform and boarded the train before we realized that we had to have our tickets punched at a machine on the platform. So the wife of the other couple and I got off the train to get the tickets punched and as we stood by the kiosk getting the tickets punched, the doors of the train closed and the train slowly left the station.

All we could do was wave to our spouses who were on their way to Kronborg Castle without us. An elderly woman recognized our distress and informed us that there would be another train to Helsingør in ten minutes. Sure enough ten minutes later we boarded another train and we were on our way. When we arrived in Helsingør our spouses were waiting for us on the platform. The little adventure ended well and gave us a tale to share with others on the trip.

Many of our fellow travelers just marveled at the fact that Muriel had had chemotherapy two days prior to our departure. She had suffered no ill effects from the Taxol and remained in high spirits throughout the trip. She, of course, had brought along a number of hats since she was once again in the process of having her hair fall out. Her bald head was displayed a couple of times to the delight of those who saw it.

The trip was wonderful but we are ready to continue with Muriel's adventure. Today was a get-things-in-order day. Muriel washed and dried clothes, and I picked up the newspapers and mail, and then mowed and raked the lawn. How does one accumulate so much mail in 16 days? Welcome home!

Wednesday, May 19, 1999

After breakfast we went to Dr. Koenig's office for Muriel's blood test. The WBC count was 6.8 and the RBC count was 4.38. Both of these were in the acceptable range. The platelet count was 446, on the high side but not critical. With everything in order Muriel was given the go-ahead for her chemotherapy session the next day. We were both suffering from jet lag, so we spent some time lazing around and trying to get our bodies back on Eastern Daylight Time.

Thursday, May 20, 1999

Muriel was scheduled for her third round of chemotherapy at 9:00 this morning and we arrived by ten to the hour. Initially she had her weight (125½ pounds) and blood pressure (164/84) measured and then saw Dr. Koenig. As he came into the room he asked, "How was your trip to Scandinavia?"

"It was great," she answered and then provided a brief summary of our trip.

"Did you experience any difficulties?"

"None whatsoever. Our fellow travelers were surprised to learn I had just had chemotherapy only two days before we left."

He then examined Muriel, and all seemed well. "You are good to go. We'll proceed with the chemotherapy."

From the examination room we walked to the chemotherapy room. As the seat in the back corner of the room was available Muriel seated herself and got comfortable. It did not take the nurse long to get her hooked up to the IV. Initially blood was drawn and then she was given Kytril. Next came Zantac, then Benadryl. At 10:05 she began with the Taxol drip, which lasted for an hour. Once more it seemed all of the precautionary medications worked their magic, because Muriel continued to suffer no ill effects from the chemotherapy. However, she again did not eat any lunch. In the afternoon Muriel curled up with another "feel good" movie while I was off to Fellowship, Fun, and Games to get my weekly bridge fix.

Thursday, May 27, 1999

Today we journeyed to Dr. Koenig's office for the weekly blood test. Both the WBC count (3.7) and the platelets (295) were below the acceptable range, but did not seem to set off any bells. There are still three weeks until the next Taxol treatment. After the blood test we stopped off at New Earth to pick up some herbal supplements that Muriel needed. Sue Wells was in the store and Muriel briefly shared about our overseas journey and her latest trip for chemotherapy. They are due to get together again with the other members of the cancer support group on the first Saturday in June.

Friday, May 28, 1999

I played golf in the morning while Muriel slept in. When she awoke she prepared her shopping list and after lunch we went grocery shopping for the month of June. As usual Muriel had her list arranged by the aisles in the store, so we were done in good order. When we returned home, we unloaded the car and put the groceries in their proper places. We then prepared to depart for Cleveland and the last concert of the year.

We again ate at China Gate Restaurant. This time I had General Tso's Chicken and Muriel had a vegetarian dish. We had the white rice and a pot of hot green tea and received the usual fortune cookies at the end of the meal. Much of the conversation for the evening was centered around the fact that in June chemotherapy will be history, and the next item on the adventure agenda was the removal of her left breast. We determined we needed to gather the letters from her doctors to send to the insurance company so the procedure could be approved.

After dinner we drove to Severance Hall to enjoy the Cleveland Orchestra. The program began with *Asyla* by Thomas Adès, followed by Ravel's Piano Concerto in G Major. Pierre-Laurent Aimard was the soloist. After the intermission we had the privilege of listening to Tchaikovsky's Symphony No. 6, *Pathétique*. There is nothing like listening to a classic orchestral piece and going home with a great feeling in your being. Even though the drive home was no shorter, the warmth of the concert and beautiful spring evening sure seemed to make it feel that way.

Thursday, June 3, 1999

After breakfast we drove to Dr. Koenig's office for Muriel to have her blood checked at 9:15. Her WBC count was at 3.3, below normal, and the platelets were at 355, above the acceptable range. Perhaps the two readings offset each other, as no alarms were sounded as Muriel prepared for her final chemotherapy session.

Thursday, June 10, 1999

It is a little hard to believe that we are driving in today for the last session of chemotherapy. What began on September 25, 1998 is coming to a close today. Muriel has endured 8 months and 16 days of differing treatments and there are no guarantees that the cancer is gone. She was scheduled for 9:30 and we arrived about ten minutes early. No matter how many times we have been to Dr. Koenig's office for blood tests or for treatment and examinations, it is always the same, overflowing with patients. Admittedly, there are three doctors in the practice, but there seems to be a never-ending supply of individuals in some stage of their struggle with cancer.

We were called into the patient preparation area where Muriel was weighed (124 pounds) and had her blood pressure taken (110/72). When Dr. Koenig came in he asked Muriel how she was doing. Muriel told him, "I think I am getting a sinus infection."

"I'll write a prescription for Cipro that will hopefully clear that up."

"Thank you. Well, today's my last chemotherapy session. Where do we go from here?" Muriel asked.

"Tamoxifen therapy if you wish to continue treatment. You would take the pill daily as adjuvant therapy."

I asked what both Muriel and I were thinking. "What does that mean?"

"After today your primary treatment will be complete. Adjuvant therapy, in this case in the form of tamoxifen, is secondary treatment. The primary treatment consisted of the mastectomy, the chemotherapy, radiation, and now more chemotherapy. Adjuvant therapy would be introduced to help prevent the development of new cancers and help prevent the return of the breast cancer. Like the other treatments you have had, you need to decide if you want to continue on this therapy."

"Why would I *not* want to do that?"

"We can discuss the pros and cons, but there is a different aim with adjuvant therapy. Until now, we have been treating your *actual* cancer. Tamoxifen therapy will be treatment for your *risk* of further cancer."

"I imagine it's a good idea to try to lower my risk."

"Yes, and that is my recommendation, but you may not *need* adjuvant therapy. After today, you could very well be cured."

"I see," Muriel said. It seemed a long moment before anyone said anything. No one in the room except God can say she is cured for certain, so planning a prophylactic mastectomy is just a preventative measure. But should we have faith that God has already cured her?

Dr. Koenig saved us from our immediate confusion as to what to do. "I don't need an answer right now. Discuss it with Keith. After treatment today, we'll give you some literature about tamoxifen to help you decide. Study it and learn about the potential side effects, and at your next appointment we'll see if you have come to a decision."

He then performed his regular examination and when completed, we moved to the chemotherapy room. The nurse easily tapped into Muriel's port and the last session was underway. Time again passed quickly, though this time rather than the distraction of reading material, we distracted ourselves as we quietly contemplated the adventures to come. I also prayed to God for His guidance. Toward the end of the session, a nurse handed me the literature about tamoxifen and told us to call if we had any questions between visits.

Before leaving we visited Dr. Flynn to discuss Muriel's progress and determine what steps were necessary to obtain the go-ahead for the surgery to remove the port and her left breast. He told us he needed the recommendation letters and he also gave us a tentative date for the surgery on the 1st of July.

As we left the office I said, "The adventure continues, but it should be all wrapped up before the first anniversary of your diagnosis." She just gave me a big grin. We were home just before lunch and Muriel chose not to eat anything. In retrospect, I suppose the pattern of Muriel's loss of appetite, specifically for lunch right after chemotherapy treatment, is the one minor side effect Muriel experienced. By dinner time each evening though, her appetite was back. Speaking of which, tonight I was scheduled to make dinner so we took it easy for the afternoon.

Tomorrow night, we will be eating out to celebrate more than one milestone.

Friday, June 11, 1999

Today is Muriel's birthday. She slept in, so I had to wait patiently until she appeared downstairs to sing "Happy Birthday" and present her with the traveling card and a gift. It is her 64th birthday and now we are the same age until I pass her by again in October.

I was a substitute in a golf league in the afternoon, and then Muriel and I went out to celebrate her birthday and the completion of all the treatments for her adventure. We drove all the way out to Montrose and had dinner at Romano's Macaroni Grill. I had the grilled pork chops with penne pasta and Muriel had a shrimp scampi dish. The server set out a big jug of wine on the table and we were on the honor system to report how many glasses we consumed. We don't usually have dessert, but they have a good tiramisu so we shared a serving. While we ate it I asked Muriel, "Do you remember the song 'When I'm Sixty-Four' by the Beatles?"

"I have a faint recollection of the melody but none of the words."

"I don't remember most of them, just the important ones."

I began to quietly sing to her, "When I get older, losing my hair, many years from now." I skipped a verse and continued, "Will you still need me, will you still feed me when I'm sixty-four?"

"I think you've had too much wine."

"Oh no, I was singing those words as if you were singing them to me, and I can tell you after 40-plus years I can answer all the questions in the affirmative."

"You're a real nut case, do you know that?"

"I know, but I love you so very much. Happy sixty-four."

Muriel is feeling great and was looking forward to continuing her life and doing some more traveling. We shared our togetherness long into the evening.

Thursday, June 17, 1999

We drove to Kent this morning as Muriel had an appointment with Dr. Waugh, her internist. This was the follow-up visit that had been recommended by Muriel's radiation oncologist when she had completed all of her radiation. She also sought Dr. Waugh's support in her decision to have a prophylactic mastectomy. He did offer his support and also agreed to prepare a letter for the insurance company. Since Muriel had completed all of her cancer treatments, after her examination he sent her to the hospital satellite to have blood drawn and various analyses performed.

This blood draw was the penultimate time Muriel was able to have a pain-free needle stick, as she also intends to have the port removed when the prophylactic mastectomy is performed. To remove the port is a gamble, because Muriel has no knowledge if her body is cancer-free. Though she did not say so explicitly, I feel that her decision to remove the port speaks to her personal faith that God has delivered her from cancer, a faith I quietly share.

< 5 >
A PROPHYLACTIC MASTECTOMY

T hursday, June 24, 1999

Dr. Flynn has taken charge of clearing Muriel's surgery with the insurance company and today I faxed him letters from Dr. Koenig, her oncologist, Dr. Walsh, her radiation oncologist, and Dr. Waugh, her internist. Dr. Flynn will use these letters, together with his own, to apprise the insurance company of the medical necessity to remove Muriel's other breast.

In addition to forwarding the letters, I called Dr. Flynn's office and ascertained that the surgery is still scheduled for the first of July. I was assured that if the insurance company responded positively the surgery will indeed be taking place as scheduled.

Monday, June 28, 1999

As a prelude to her anticipated surgery, after lunch we went to the hospital so Muriel could pre-register and take care of the pre-admission testing ordered by Dr. Flynn. One of the procedures was a mammogram that to me seemed unnecessary since she was due to have the breast removed on Thursday. However, it is apparently one of the tests administered prior to a mastectomy. If indeed there is evidence of cancer, the excision may have to be different than a normal mastectomy.

After the completion of the mammogram we crossed the bridge on the second level of the hospital and went to the outpatient hematology laboratory where Muriel was to have her blood drawn. It will be the last time she will be able to use the port and undergo an essentially pain-free blood draw. The WBC count (7.7), the RBC count (4.79), and the platelets (371) were all in the acceptable ranges. There do not appear to be any hindrances to proceeding with the surgery on Thursday.

We made our way home and enjoyed lunch. Late in the afternoon the phone rang. Muriel answered and after a brief conversation turned to me and said, "That was Dr. Flynn's office. Mutual approved the surgery so it's a go for Thursday."

Echoing a sentiment I had shared before, I added, "The adventure continues."

Thursday, July 1, 1999

Muriel was scheduled for surgery at 10:00. This trip for a mastectomy seemed so different from the first trip in September of last year. Our children had been routinely informed and a report to them would be after the fact as Muriel was essentially undergoing "preventative maintenance." We arrived at the hospital a little after 9:00. Muriel went to the surgery prep area and changed into a hospital gown. All of her clothes were folded and put into a plastic bag and given to me. The last item, as usual, was her glasses. She told me later that before she went to surgery she had a chest X-ray. Apparently Dr. Flynn wanted to know the exact location of the port.

I retired to the surgical waiting room and reported to the volunteer in charge where I would be sitting in the event Dr. Flynn needed to be in touch with me. Since it was my second time around in the surgery waiting room, I was less aware of the comings and goings of other persons. Since this surgery was not life threatening, no pastor and no friends came by to offer support. I was still feeling the peace from God that Muriel had prayed for nearly ten months ago. I spent time reading and soon I was being paged to speak with Dr. Flynn. All had gone well with Muriel's operation, including the removal of the port. He told me she was in the recovery room and welcomed me to go sit with her.

I immediately went to the recovery room and the nurse on duty directed me to the bed where Muriel was recovering. She was still under the influence of the anesthesia.

She began to rouse about 45 minutes after my arrival. Her first words again were, "May I have my glasses?"

I laughed and held them out to her and she quickly slipped them on. "I love you," I said, bending over to give her a kiss. She was quite groggy but still managed to say, "I love you too, but now I'll never be Mrs. America."

I laughed again as she grinned, slowly closing her eyes. I said, "You'll always be *my* Mrs. America." I kissed her again gently on the forehead and held her hand as she continued to become more lucid. An hour later she was ready to go to her room, so I accompanied her as she was transported by gurney to the oncology wing of the hospital and her semi-private room.

I judged it best that she rest, so I departed to tend to some things at home and have dinner. I returned to the hospital and found Muriel to be in good spirits. She was eating dinner and surprisingly appeared to be relishing it. It was definitely not a bland meal this time. She swallowed a bite and said excitedly, "I slept for a while after you left and when I woke up I just said all sorts of prayers thanking God for everything, the two successful surgeries, the chemotherapy without nausea, the radiation, having the port put in, and even for the loss of my hair."

I was excited as well. "God's peace has certainly carried the day for you. I am so proud of how you've handled everything and it's been a pleasure to be at your side, though you're the one who did all of the heavy lifting."

"No, we did it together, with the help of God. Thank you sweetie for all you've done to help me through this adventure. I love you so much."

"I love you too."

Even though she was in the middle of eating her dinner, we hugged and kissed as tears trickled down our cheeks. While Muriel continued her dinner we sustained our conversation. When she was finished, we held hands and prayed that the removal of the other breast would clear the final hurdle to a full recovery. She added a final exclamation point to the conversation saying, "I never have to wear a bra again!" As the evening wore on and Muriel started to tire, we agreed that I would return home and await her call in the morning as to when I should pick her up. I gave her a kiss goodnight and departed.

Friday, July 2, 1999

Muriel called about 9:30 to tell me she would be ready to come home at 11:00. I had finished my exercises by the time she had called so I showered and left right away to go to the bank, drop off the water bill payment, get stamps, and pick up a new battery for my watch. I still managed to arrive just before 11:00. I had parked the car in the emergency room parking lot, so after Muriel received going-home instructions she got into a wheelchair and the nurse took her down to the discharge area by the ER.

I moved the car into position and helped Muriel get seated, belting her into the passenger seat. She was feeling very chipper, but we decided not to go to the Blossom Music Center where we were scheduled to hear the Cleveland Orchestra. Muriel seemed to be content to eat pizza for dinner, so I called Pizza Hut and ordered a medium pizza with pepperoni and mushrooms. On my way to pick up the pizza I dropped off a prescription for hydrocodone to be used to reduce any pain that might arise. So our fare for the evening was pizza and beer. She had three slices and was sated. I could have eaten all of the rest, but I saved three slices in the event she wanted to have some for lunch on Saturday.

Sunday, July 4, 1999

It is the first Sunday of the month, so we went to the first service where we were able to take Communion and thank God for all the blessings that He has given to Muriel during her adventure. Public prayers were said for Muriel for the successful surgery. At the end of the service many of our fellow parishioners came by to give Muriel a hug and wish her well as she moved forward with her life. It is generally at those times when people ask me how I am doing. I am always a little embarrassed, because the peace which Muriel had prayed for seems to continue to envelop her life and just catches me up in it. So I can only respond that I am doing great, which is a testament to how God is working not only in Muriel's life, but in my life as well.

Wednesday, July 7, 1999

Muriel had an appointment to see Dr. Koenig today. It has been approximately one month since she had her last dose of Taxol. She went through the usual routine: got weighed (124 pounds), had her blood pressure taken (130/70), and was examined by Dr. Koenig.

"How are you feeling?" he asked.

"I'm feeling great and I think I'd like to proceed with taking the tamoxifen, but I'd like to know more about the side effects."

"Sure thing. Did you read the literature Beth gave you?"

"Yes, hot flashes, headaches, and fatigue I can take, but it also mentioned potential for blood clots, strokes, and uterine cancer?"

"Those more serious side effects are a lot less common. Studies have shown that there have been occurrences of blood clots, strokes, and even uterine cancer, but the percentage over the normal occurrence is really quite small."

"Well, I have managed all right with the treatments thus far, so maybe my luck will continue."

"You've done better than all right. You've done great. And the studies have firmly established that the benefits far outweigh the potential risks. Do you still think you'd like to proceed with the tamoxifen therapy? If you aren't ready to decide you can have more time."

"No, I think I'm ready. Let's do it."

Muriel received a starting sample of the pills and a prescription to allow us to get a 90-day supply. We made an appointment to see Dr. Koenig in four months. With the pills to help ward off future cancers, we judge the adventure is winding down.

Thursday, July 8, 1999

Today marks the one-week anniversary of Muriel's second mastectomy, and we went to see Dr. Flynn to have her dressing changed and the drainage tube removed. During the week we have been very faithful at stripping the tubing and recording the cc of fluid we removed. Dr. Flynn was very pleased with the healing process and removed the drainage tube and redressed the incision.

Friday, July 9, 1999

This evening we went to Porthouse Theatre, which is located on the grounds of the Blossom Music Center, the summer home of the Cleveland Orchestra. We saw Shakespeare's *Much Ado About Nothing*. What a treat it was for Muriel. She has been a Shakespeare buff since high school and Shakespeare, unbeknownst to him, had been one of the moving forces that prompted her to change her major after her freshman year at Trenton State College from music to English. She then got an M.A. in English at the University of Akron and immediately began teaching there part time. Every year she taught freshman composition, she would have her students read and discuss one of Shakespeare's plays. In spite of all the papers she had to correct, the times she taught the Shakespeare portion of the course was just a touch of nirvana.

The first trip we ever took overseas, sponsored by *National Geographic*, was to England where we were privileged to visit Stratford-on-Avon. We saw the house where Shakespeare was born and visited Holy Trinity Church where he was buried. He had the honor to be buried in the chancel and there is a monument on the wall nearest his grave that features a bust showing him posed in the act of writing. Each year at the time of his birthday a new quill pen is placed in the writing hand of the bust.

Muriel was emotionally overcome and cried when we visited the church and the grave site of Shakespeare. It was just a very special day for her. Thus, on this day to be in the audience where one of Shakespeare's plays was being performed brought back all of the wonderful memories she has of her associations with William Shakespeare and the plays he had written.

Monday, July 19, 1999

We were back to Dr. Flynn's office again this morning so Muriel could have her stitches checked and the dressing removed. Dr. Flynn was very pleased with the progress of the healing and released Muriel with a clean bill of health. The dressing was greatly reduced and we will not be required to make any additional visits. Though there are of course no guarantees, to me this surely feels like the end of the adventure.

Saturday, July 24, 1999

Today I drove Muriel to the airport where she boarded a flight to Texas to visit her sister, Judith, and her husband, Richard. She will also be seeing our children and grandchildren while she is there. Muriel and her sister have been exchanging visits for several years. They had not always been that close, as their parents seemed to play them off against each other. However, they finally decided that they were tired of playing games and as adults united in an effort to halt the pettiness that had been created by their parents.

At that time, Judith and Richard were living in Endwell, New York and Muriel would drive up one year and Judith would drive to Ohio the next. Then Richard's company relocated him to Texas and they bought a home in Arlington, a suburb of Dallas. So whenever we go to Texas to see our family, we always spend some time with Judith and Richard. It is a little more difficult for Judith to come visit Muriel. What added to the difficulty is the fact that Judith had a bout with scleroderma and then had kidney problems that ultimately led to her being on dialysis. Judith too had had breast cancer and had her right breast removed, and she also went through chemotherapy and radiation therapy as well. However, Judith chose to have reconstructive breast surgery which enabled her to forgo wearing a prosthesis. Muriel, on the other hand, is happy to be sans breasts. At least that is what she tells me.

While she is in Texas, both of our kids and their families will make the trip to Arlington to visit Oma, the name Muriel had elected from the German for grandmother. I have been, and will continue to be, Grandpa rather than Opa, the name some men of German descent have chosen.

< 6 >
THE REST OF 1999

Monday, August 2, 1999

This afternoon I picked Muriel up at Cleveland Hopkins International Airport as she was returning from Texas. I was waiting for her when she came down Concourse C. She looked terrific and I gave her a big hug and kiss. We walked hand in hand to the baggage area where I picked up her luggage and we continued on to the car. We stopped in Macedonia on the return trip home and ate dinner at the Ground Round. I got to hear all about her days in Texas and particularly about our grandchildren. She had had a very nice visit with her sister, marking the first time they had been together since Muriel's adventure had begun. It is great that they had the opportunity to share some quality time together.

Friday, August 13, 1999

We had packed the car yesterday, and this morning we left for home after a week's stay in North Myrtle Beach. It was about a 12-hour drive for us but we had started early enough so that we arrived in Munroe Falls around 5:00, driving straight through to our home with the usual complement of potty, gas, and lunch breaks.

South Carolina had been wonderful. We had a time-share week at Fairfield Westwinds, a high-rise building right on the ocean. We stayed in a two-bedroom condominium with two baths, a living/dining room that also contained a hide-a-bed, and a full kitchen. We spent the week with our daughter Kay and her two children. We had predetermined that Kay would cook three meals and that Muriel or I would cook three meals, and we would go out for the buffet at one of the many Calabash restaurants for our 7th meal.

Muriel had brought along her usual seven books for a weekly time-share, and she and Kaitlyn spent time on the beach soaking up the sun and dipping their feet in the ocean. Muriel was only a little over a month removed from her surgery and could go in the water only up to her thighs. However, it was enough to be exhilarating and therapeutic for her. Kay, Kenton, and I spent the mornings playing several of the wonderful golf courses on the Grand Strand and in the afternoons enjoyed the ocean. In the evenings, we all played our ongoing games of UNO or Phase 10, or we assembled pieces of the 1,000-piece jigsaw puzzle that I had brought. Everyone had a great time and the week went by much too fast. After we unpacked the car, I picked up a pizza for dinner as we relaxed and reminisced about the week at the beach.

Friday, September 3, 1999

Over the rest of August we began to settle into the routines we had accustomed ourselves to before the adventure began. I played golf on Mondays and Wednesdays and we played together on Fridays. Muriel had begun to resume all of the duties around the home that she had done previously, such as washing and ironing and taking care of the meals. We agreed to have a house cleaner come in once a month to do all of the vacuuming and dusting. That was a gift to me, since I was the one who had routinely done those tasks.

Muriel attended her support group which met once a month. As the person in charge of humor, she went all out to make sure she had material that would elicit laughter, though the group returned the favor. Since it was the first support group meeting she had attended since her second mastectomy, she was presented with a T-shirt emblazoned with "AS IS" across the front of it. She wore it proudly.

We went to church and Sunday School on Sundays. We continued our activities with Stephen Ministry. We are both members of the planning committee at church and Muriel is also part of the Board of Human Care, serving as its initial chairperson. We went out to dinner and attended Cleveland Orchestra concerts at the Blossom Music Center. Life is good and the cancer is behind us.

Saturday, September 4, 1999

"We did it," I cheered.

"Did you expect differently?" Muriel asked, grinning widely.

I grinned back just as widely. This was a re-enactment of sorts of the scene played out last October when Muriel and I completed our first hike after her first surgery.

"Don't you owe me a kiss?" she asked, still grinning.

"Of course. Here's to many more," I said as I kissed and hugged her. In all honesty, I wasn't certain we would have earned our medallions this year, but here we are again with eight hikes under our belts.

Wednesday, November 3, 1999

We settled further into our normal routines during September and October. Muriel continues to be back to full health and is enjoying her life to the fullest. She looks great and has no problem being without breasts. Her hair is back and seems to be even curlier than before the chemotherapy. We renewed our tickets to the Cleveland Orchestra concerts even though we had debated not doing it. We also renewed our tickets to the Akron Symphony Orchestra concerts. In addition, selected shows from the offerings at E. J. Thomas Hall and the three performances of Ohio Ballet provided us a full slate of the arts. We went on to hike most of our 13 trails, finishing up in October and adding another medallion to our walking sticks.

In October I spent more time raking leaves than mowing the lawn. On the 20th of the month we began our journey to Hawaii. It was primarily a cruise and we picked up the ship after flying to Oahu. The first few days were spent in Honolulu where we went to Pearl Harbor and out to the USS *Arizona* Memorial. It was a very solemn occasion. Some free time afforded us the opportunity to buy ourselves some Hawaiian outfits for shipboard Hawaiian activities. Muriel got a blue print dress with appliquéd designs and I got a matching shirt. I also picked up another tropical shirt later in the trip. We spent some time at Waikiki Beach and watched the surfers. Our itinerary included a bus trip to the Polynesian Cultural Center where we saw exhibits and demonstrations by natives from the different Polynesian islands. The day culminated in an enjoyable luau. We also visited the Foster Botanical Garden.

Our ship then took us to the "Big Island," Hawaii, where we stopped on the eastern side at Hilo and then traveled across the island to the western side at Kona. We made an interesting discovery at Kona. We found a restaurant named Pancho and Lefty's. Back home in Ohio in the village of Stow there is also a Pancho and Lefty's, so we picked up a menu to share with the Ohio location. We also visited the famous Parker Ranch in Waimea.

The next stop was Maui. Time was spent in Lahaina. We saw the huge banyan tree that was planted in 1873 and is nearly the size of a city block. That is a lot of shade. We lunched at the Bubba Gump Shrimp Co. restaurant of *Forrest Gump* fame. We next visited the island of Kauai and took the riverboat up the Wailua River to visit Fern Grotto. It is a natural amphitheater with ferns growing out of what is essentially the roof. There was a trio there playing Hawaiian music and the acoustics were just great.

Because our cruise had originated in the Hawaiian islands it was necessary to cruise to a set of islands that were not part of America to accommodate some arcane rules of the sea, though I do not recall where it was that we stopped. On our way a woman aboard had an appendicitis and had to be airlifted from the ship. Thus, our ship had to turn around and meet the life flight at its range point. As a result we lost a day and never did get to Lanai. Throughout the trip we encountered an ABC Store on nearly every street corner as well as numerous Hilo Hatties. The cruise company was terrific and we took all sorts of pictures. The food was good and the sightseeing was great. Our cruise ended back on Oahu. Yesterday we flew out of Honolulu and returned to Ohio, and today we were welcomed back to the real world by going to see Dr. Walsh, the radiation oncologist. It was Muriel's six-month check-up since the completion of the radiation therapy. Dr. Walsh was pleased with her progress and said she had no irregularities due to the radiation. She made an appointment for further follow-up in six months.

Thursday, November 11, 1999

Muriel had a follow-up appointment with Dr. Koenig this morning. His office was very busy, as usual, and we waited our turn to be called by the nurse. Initially Muriel was weighed (125 pounds) and then had her blood pressure taken (132/78) before Dr. Koenig entered.

"How are you?" he asked.

"I'm doing very well. That prescription for Hawaii was some good medicine," she answered. The three of us laughed, then she added, "I do think the tamoxifen therapy may be giving me some hot flashes and night sweats, but overall I'm feeling really good."

"Great. Let's see how you're doing." He examined her fully and upon completion he suggested she have a full liver panel function. "If we do this periodically, any reoccurrence of the cancer would be able to be detected."

"Do you think the cancer has returned?" Muriel asked.

"No, no, but just as we were aggressive toward the cancer in the beginning, we want to use all means to keep apprised of the way your body is reacting as we move forward."

We left the examination room and stepped into the blood draw area. After getting squared away in a chair I held Muriel's hand, as she was now going to experience her first needle stick without benefit of a port in over a year. The technician was quite adept and found a vein without any difficulty. When the draw was complete I made an appointment to return in four months and we departed. As we walked to the car Muriel said, "I think he wants to be precautionary."

I said, "Precautionary is good." We left it at that and returned home.

Saturday, November 13, 1999

We got a call from Dr. Koenig's office yesterday to inform Muriel that there had been a lab accident and that the hepatic function panel needed to be redrawn. I checked with Muriel and it was her decision to wait until she returned to his office in March of 2000 to have it done then. I judge that Muriel is attempting to exert a little control in her life and she will be the arbiter of when she will have a blood draw. Then again, she just may have not wanted to have another needle stick.

Tonight we went out to dinner and then to the Akron Civic Theatre where we enjoyed a concert by pianist George Winston. Although he is somewhat minimalist in his playing, he does have some very nice original pieces.

Friday, December 31, 1999

We spent the vast majority of the rest of 1999 traveling. On Wednesday, November 17th, we left for Texas and ultimately on to Pagosa Springs, Colorado where we spent the Thanksgiving weekend with Kay and her family. Kay, just like last year, brought along a smoked turkey and ham which made for a delicious Thanksgiving dinner. It was anticipated that we would be able to ski, but alas, there was no snow on the mountain. So we filled some of the time by going to Mesa Verde National Park. This national park offers a spectacular look into the history of the ancestral Pueblo people who lived there for over 700 years. Because of the good weather, we were able to visit some of the cliff dwellings which were unbelievably well-preserved. We had the benefit of a park ranger who guided us through the dwellings. We were able to tick off another of the 1,000 places to see before you die. However, I don't think we are going to see all 1,000 of them before God calls us home.

Our evenings were filled with more UNO and Phase 10 games as well as working on the jigsaw puzzle that Kay brought. However, that puzzle was 2,000 pieces and depicted the inside of a cathedral, and was just a very difficult puzzle. Even with several of us working on it, it did not get completed. I packed it up and brought it back to Ohio where I can work on it in my leisure.

Kay and her family packed up and returned to Dallas on the Sunday after Thanksgiving. I had booked two additional time-share weeks in Pagosa Springs, with the intent that I would drive to Wolf Creek for some time on the slopes. I did finally get to ski on the last two days of the three-week stay, albeit only the bunny slopes were open. Wolf Creek is noted year after year for getting the most snow on their slopes in all of Colorado. The year 1999 was the exception.

Kay had left us with all of the leftover food, so we had turkey with all of the trimmings as well as a honey-baked ham. We had brought coffee and cereal and other staples, so eating was not a problem. I had included one 1,000-piece puzzle which I completed in short order. As the first week progressed, Muriel and I also read all of the books we had brought so it gave us a reason to drive to Durango fifty miles west of Pagosa Springs. Another reason to go to Durango was the fact that I thought I had heard something on TV that had said there was still skiing at Purgatory. I was eager to ski but that lead turned out to be incorrect, a TV mirage likely due to my wishful thinking. I suppose right then if someone had said "There's no way down Wolf Creek" I would have heard "There's snow way down Wolf Creek."

While in Durango, we walked the historic streets and visited the railroad museum. On our return to Pagosa Springs we stopped at a K-Mart where we picked up some books and three more puzzles. We had an enjoyable two weeks, and Muriel is moving on with her life in a cancer-free manner.

We returned from Colorado on December 17th with just enough time to wash our clothes, sort through the mail, and get ready for Christmas and our trip to New Bern, North Carolina. During the week, I had an appointment with my urologist, we picked up supplements at New Earth, went to Chorale practice, and sang on Christmas Eve. After the Christmas Eve service we had our usual spread consisting of shrimp, several cheeses, beef sticks, a variety of crackers, and some hot hors d'oeuvres. Together with a glass of White Zinfandel, we snacked and shared our Christmas presents.

On the 26th of December we left for our trip to New Bern, staying right on the inlet at our time-share at Fairfield Harbour. We soaked up the sun and continued to count our blessings that all is proceeding in good order regarding Muriel's adventure. We will ring in the New Year in New Bern tonight and, after spending one more day here, we will make our way to Virginia for the next leg of our trip.

< 7 >
NEW TWISTS AND TURNS IN 2000

Sunday, January 2, 2000

We departed from New Bern, North Carolina and drove up Route 17 toward Virginia. After crossing into Williamston the route turned to the east, and we essentially drove across the north side of Albemarle Sound, a very scenic route. Just before you get to the Atlantic Ocean, the route once again turned to the north and carried us into Virginia. We picked up I-64 and then I-264 which took us directly to Virginia Beach, where we had a second time-share week booked. We were right on the beach, and although it definitely was not swimming weather, we looked forward to oceanside walks on the boardwalk.

Friday, January 7, 2000

We packed the car in anticipation of our departure from Virginia in the morning. The time-share facilities had been minimal and doing a 1,000-piece puzzle on a circular table that did not hold all of the pieces proved to be a challenge, but it was a nice quiet week with walks on the beach and the boardwalk outside, and reading and puzzling inside. We also took the opportunity to reflect on the adventure and where we are in the scheme of things. We concluded that Dr. Koenig had taken a very aggressive approach to the treatment of Muriel's cancer and that all is well.

"Three more years," Muriel said.

"What do you mean?"

"If I get through the next three years I will be free and clear of this cancer. If it comes back it won't be because of the breast cancer." So the whole approach to this new year is to move forward as if the cancer is overcome and we have the rest of our lives in front of us.

Wednesday, January 12, 2000

We had returned home on the 8th of January, and today Muriel had an appointment with Dr. Karlen, her gynecological oncologist. She had a pelvic examination which included a Pap smear. There was no immediate indication of any problems.

Tonight while we ate dinner I noticed Muriel would soon need another haircut. We have continued to work on her hair since it had grown back, and I now have the privilege of cutting it on a regular basis. To ensure that I don't make a mess of it, I make little snips in one section and then we get the hand mirror for Muriel to check that I have not done anything drastic. With each successive haircut we go longer between views with the mirror as I got the hang of how she wanted to have it look. I'm not sure whether the professional hairdressers have difficulty with hair that is really curly or if it makes it easier to cut. In any event, I find the waves to be helpful in guiding me as I cut on the turn of the hair from one wave to the next. That way I had some basis for holding the hair between my fingers and making a cut. The haircuts are win-win propositions. I enjoy cutting her hair, she likes the results, and we are afforded more opportunities to enjoy one another's company.

Saturday, January 22, 2000

Today was "wash the sheets and make the beds" day. That is one of the duties around the house that I regularly did even before Muriel's adventure. Muriel slept in until 11:00 and it wasn't until after lunch that I had completed my tasks. In the evening we went to Applebee's and then on to E. J. Thomas Hall where we enjoyed another concert by the Akron Symphony Orchestra. The concert began with the Saint-Saëns Violin Concerto No. 3 in B Minor, Op. 5 with Chee-Yun as the featured violinist. The program also included the Overture to *Rienzi* by Wagner and Symphony No. 5 in D Major by Ralph Vaughan Williams. The concert was under the direction of Harry Davidson. He was another of the candidates on review to fill the role of music director after the loss of Alan Balter, who had died of cancer before the start of the new concert season. We left the concert in an upbeat mood, but hurried to our car in the frigid weather and were home in ten minutes.

Thursday, January 27, 2000

Today Muriel was to see Dr. Daniel Abood, her new general practitioner. Dr. Waugh, who had taken care of both of us, had retired at the end of 1999, and it was necessary for each of us to find a new GP. I had elected to have Dr. Pennie Marchetti as my GP but Muriel did not want to have a woman doctor. Dr. Waugh had sold his practice to Dr. Abood and Muriel elected to utilize his services. His office was located in Kent, but was a little closer to home than Dr. Waugh's office. Muriel has been suffering from what she deemed to be a sinus infection. She has also experienced intermittent shortness of breath and wanted to have him deal with that as well.

Upon entering Dr. Abood's office we were greeted by Dottie, Dr. Waugh's nurse who had accompanied the turnover of the practice. It was nice to see a familiar face in this unfamiliar place. Dottie brought Muriel into an examination room and recorded her blood pressure (110/80), weight (124 pounds), temperature (98.6°) and pulse (80). Dottie departed and we awaited the entry of Muriel's new GP. Before long Dr. Abood entered and introduced himself, shaking hands with each of us. He appeared to be of Indian descent and looked to be in his thirties. He exuded a sense of confidence and there was an immediate comfortableness with his manner. Muriel began by presenting her list of medications which he scanned without comment. He then asked, "Why are you here today?"

"I think I should bring you up to date on my recent medical history." Muriel explained all about the two mastectomies, the chemotherapy and radiation treatments, and that she is now on tamoxifen therapy. Lastly she said, "I think I have a sinus infection and I'm also experiencing shortness of breath, and I've been experiencing frequent bowel movements with pains in my abdomen, some very severe."

"I'm sorry you're experiencing all of this discomfort. Let's see if we can do something about it." He asked many questions and gave her a thorough examination. "I want you to have a chest X-ray, a complete blood work-up, and pulmonary tests to better help me address the difficulties you are experiencing. I also recommend that you visit a gastroenterologist regarding your abdominal pain. He will probably want to do a colonoscopy, which I would also recommend."

We thanked him for his concern, and as we departed he left her with the order requisitions for all of the tests he had recommended and provided her with four prescriptions to relieve her discomfort:

Zithromax for her sinus infection, and albuterol, Atrovent, and Flonase to help her with her breathing. We stopped at CVS on the way home to drop off the prescriptions and I picked them up later in the day.

Friday, January 28, 2000

This morning we returned to Kent to the outpatient clinic associated with Robinson Memorial Hospital, which is located in Ravenna, Ohio. I could not accompany Muriel to her blood draw but as Muriel told me later, the nurse had a gentle manner that made the experience nearly pain free. After the blood draw we walked to another part of the building for the X-ray. After completing the tests we stopped off at Dr. Abood's office and picked up two more prescriptions to help her breathing, Combivent and Flovent.

I told Muriel, "With six new prescriptions your body is going to be a walking drugstore."

She retorted, "But most of them are just to help my breathing."

"I know sweetheart, I was just yanking your chain."

We stopped at K-Mart on the way home and just looked around to see if there were any bargains. No such luck. After lunch I went to Boston Mills and skied until four while Muriel relaxed with a book.

Sunday, January 30, 2000

This is the fifth Sunday of the month and Communion is offered in both services, so we elected to go to the second service. It had snowed overnight so our late departure gave me plenty of time to shovel the driveway and sidewalks. After church, we spent a quiet day together and in the evening celebrated our 41st anniversary with the reading of our shared anniversary card and our traditional anniversary dinner, Duckling Rosé with wild rice and asparagus and a glass of rosé wine leftover from the basting process. As usual we had pecan pie for dessert.

During dinner, as she raised her glass for a toast, Muriel said, "We are now one year closer to our 50th wedding anniversary."

I raised my glass and responded, "I think we can do that. Happy anniversary. I love you."

"I love you too."

Tuesday, February 1, 2000

This morning we were on our way to Ravenna to visit Robinson Memorial Hospital. Muriel was scheduled to have several tests in regards to her breathing problems. I was not permitted to accompany her, so I found a chair in the waiting area and brought out my reading material to bide my time. After about two hours all of the tests had been completed. On the way home we stopped at GNC where we picked up several antioxidants that we used on a daily basis.

Wednesday, February 2, 2000

I ran several errands, cleared the snow from the driveway and sidewalks, made fresh bread, and began preparation for our trip to Colonial Williamsburg. Muriel put the finishing touches on a presentation she was to give in the evening. Sue Wells, the organizer of the breast cancer support group, had arranged to have a panel of some breast cancer survivors speak to a group of persons at her church. Muriel was one of three women on the panel, so after dinner we drove to the church. Each of the women provided the basic facts of their encounter with cancer and its effects on their lives. All three encouraged the women present to get a mammogram on a regular basis, as well as to speak to their doctors about self-examination. There were at least 35 persons present, most of them women. I sat with Carol Wheeler, a regular member of the support group.

Muriel was the second of the three panelists to speak and exuded confidence as she walked to the podium. Her at-ease demeanor, borne from many years of teaching, was evident. But I was certain she was also experiencing the peace that God had bestowed on her at the outset of this adventure. She gazed out at us with a wide and beautiful smile and began. "Thank you. All of you. Thank you for joining us here tonight as we each share our individual experiences with breast cancer. And I especially thank God for the peace He has given me throughout what I call my adventure with breast cancer. He truly does answer our prayers."

Muriel then proceeded to recount her adventure, never forgetting the faith that carried her, the faith that allowed her to soar above this storm. I struggled in vain to fight back the tears that welled in my eyes and joined in the applause when Muriel finished. It truly was an inspirational experience for me, and I would say, many others. Carol gave me a gentle nudge in the ribs as we clapped.

Thursday, February 3, 2000

A brand new doctor entered Muriel's life today, as if we don't have enough already. We drive one town over to Cuyahoga Falls and the Greater Akron Gastroenterology office of Dr. Michael Cline. Muriel's periodic pain in the abdomen, severe at times, was to be investigated. I did not accompany her into the examination room. When Muriel returned to the waiting area we got our coats and left. On the way to the car I asked her what happened.

"He did a thorough examination and he suggested that I have a colonoscopy. He's going to set it up and let me know."

"That's also what Dr. Abood had suggested," I replied.

Saturday, February 12, 2000

Tonight we returned home after a week-long stay in Williamsburg, Virginia. If you have never spent time in Williamsburg, I would highly recommend that you do. We had a time-share week with Fairfield and stayed at the Governor's Green. As we are wont to do, we had taken along meals for the week and just picked up the staples that we needed for our stay. We went to the historic village three different days and had a thoroughly enjoyable time. Every trip began at the visitor center where we browsed the shops and purchased our tickets. As you can imagine, the number of persons at the village was minimal given the season, so we had plenty of time to closely observe all of the homes and historic buildings. In the Randolph House there was a vintage piano that Muriel had the privilege of playing. I suspect that was not a part of the general tour. We were also able to view some historic prescription books in the apothecary. We spent time viewing the Wythe House, the Governor's Palace, the Capitol, and all of the other places along Gloucester Street.

One evening we dined at Christiana Campbell's Tavern and another we spent listening to an organ recital at the Brunton Parish Church. We checked out all of the stores in Merchant's Square, as well as the Public Hospital of 1773 and the newly constructed museum. One day we drove down to the Jamestown Settlement, and spent another in Newport News where we toured the Mariner's Museum and the Chrysler Museum of Art. Of course no trip to Williamsburg would be complete if one did not go to the Pottery Factory, so we spent a half day checking out all of the items they had to sell. I don't think I have ever seen a larger variety of dried and silk flowers, ferns, herbs, and whatever else one fancied of the inert variety. We enjoyed ourselves immensely.

Tuesday, February 15, 2000

This morning Muriel was in the hospital to have a colonoscopy. It was scheduled for 10:00 and all went well. We were out of there a bit before noon. Apparently there were no untoward problems with her bowel as we received no report of any difficulty.

Wednesday, February 16, 2000

We began the day by going to Dr. Abood's office to pick up an order requisition for Muriel to have a CT scan. Then it was on to Robinson

Memorial Hospital for her to have the actual scan. I was unable to accompany Muriel into the test area so I retreated to the waiting room while she had the test. We were home just after lunch time and watched one of Muriel's "feel good" movies.

Friday, February 18, 2000

After a light snow overnight I had the privilege of shoveling the drive and sidewalks. I think perhaps it is time to look for a condo and let someone else do such work. In the evening we drove to Cleveland for a Cleveland Orchestra concert, stopping in Macedonia at the Outback Steakhouse for dinner. Muriel had the petite steak with grilled veggies and a baked potato. I also had the grilled veggies but chose the T-bone steak with garlic mashed potatoes. Muriel had a glass of White Zinfandel and I had a 22-ounce glass of Foster's. After dinner we continued to Severance Hall and the concert. Christoph Eschenbach was the guest conductor and selected a wonderful program that began with Radu Lupu on solo piano performing Mozart's Piano Concerto No. 23 in A Major, K. 488. Then came Mahler's *Blumine* and, to end the evening, his Symphony No. 1. The Symphony was over an hour in length but ended the evening on a great high.

Saturday, March 4, 2000

It seems like our lives are back in order and Muriel is carrying on as a cancer-free person. She has been regularly attending her support group on the first Saturday of the month and shares with me the ebb and flow of the group as new people join and others depart. However, the original nucleus remains intact and they have all continued to enjoy the positive support they offer each other.

For us, back to normal entails travel, and this morning marked the beginning of our next travel chapter, a trip to Texas for our expanded family photo. We had our bags packed and left early in the morning. Of late, our drives to Texas take us through St. Louis and Springfield, Missouri, and then a short westward drive into Oklahoma before turning south for a straight shot into Texas. Since we planned on staying overnight in Joplin, Missouri at the end of the first day of driving, we did not have to leave before daylight.

Sunday, March 5, 2000

We arrived in Texas midafternoon Sunday and made accommodations at the Comfort Inn & Suites in Plano. We then went to Mark's house where we had pizza and beer. We got reacquainted with Emma and I had the privilege of playing games with her. With Emma, playing games means Emma wins. However, she didn't bargain on having a very competitively-oriented grandfather who also likes to win!

Monday, March 6, 2000

We were scheduled today to have our family picture taken. I have tried to have a family photograph done every five years. In that time frame there are definitely large changes in individuals, especially the grandchildren. This year would also mark the first time that Emma would be in the picture. She was a little antsy but we managed to get pictures of the whole family and each of the individual families. We also had photos taken of Grandpa and Oma with the grandchildren and then with our children. After the picture-taking session we all went out to eat at Maggioni's thanks to Kay's husband Larry. The restaurant is noted for its family-style dinners so we had several appetizers and then a main dish of salmon and a second of lasagna. We each had a salad and we shared a couple of bottles of Woodbridge Chardonnay. It was a pleasant time for us all.

Tuesday, March 21, 2000

We arrived home tonight after extending our vacation in Colorado for 11 days. Muriel and I, together with Kay and her family, headed there when school let out on Wednesday, March 8th. We stayed overnight in Witchita Falls, then arrived on Thursday close to dinnertime in Pagosa Springs where they had rented a house for four days. The main living room was large and circular and had a potbellied stove-type fireplace right in the center of the room. Larry began a fire as soon as we arrived that exuded warmth to all parts of the room. The room was huge, encompassing the kitchen and dining area as well. We enjoyed the remainder of the week, going to the slopes three times and in the evening playing games and working on the jigsaw puzzle Kay had brought. On Sunday, when Kay and her family headed back to Texas, Muriel and I moved to a Fairfield facility for an additional week in Pagosa Springs. Since we had driven down we brought enough books and puzzles to keep us busy. Kay provided us with some leftover food and we went to City Market to get whatever else we needed. It had been a happy, healing trip but we were glad to be home with our updated family photos in hand to mark the gathering.

Thursday, March 23, 2000

It was another drive to Kent this morning as Muriel was due to see Dr. Abood for her one month follow-up. Dottie collected Muriel's vital information: weight (134 pounds), blood pressure (120/80), temperature

(98°), and pulse (80). Dr. Abood entered the examination room as Dottie departed. He opened her folder and said, "I have the results of your colonoscopy, your CT scan, your blood work, and the chest X-ray that you had and there is nothing of consequence to report. Have all the breathing aids been helpful for your shortness of breath?"

Muriel said, "There has definitely been some improvement in my breathing."

I added, "She maintains a notebook and records the specific type of inhaler each time she uses one."

"Has there been any change in the occurrence of your hot flashes?"

"I haven't had as many but I'm still having them."

The doctor then proceeded with a thorough examination. When he was done he said, "I'm going to give you a prescription for Bellergal-S which should help you with your hot flashes." He also provided us with new prescriptions for Flovent and Combivent.

Monday, March 27, 2000

After lunch today, we returned to Kent where Muriel was scheduled to undergo a bone density test. While Muriel had her test, I took the opportunity to reflect on her adventure. In my mind I likened it to one's general attitude toward the weather, particularly for those of us who live in the northern hemisphere where the winter months seem to drag on and on and on. Finally there is spring and the temperatures begin to creep up and ultimately we reach the high 70s and low 80s. At that point we forget all about those winter months, having no remembrance of how many days we had with subzero temperatures and how many inches of snow we had for the year. It is all behind us. That seems to be the picture of Muriel. The long ordeal of chemotherapy, then radiation, then chemotherapy again, all of the tests and blood draws, two surgeries, they were all behind her. But now, just like in spring when some days are marred with rain and thundershowers, her life is interrupted by CT scans, bone density exams, and more blood draws. The snow, the cold, the extended darkness of winter were behind her and her life turned mostly to sunshine and warmth. The bone density test was over in an hour and we returned home.

Thursday, March 30, 2000

Today Muriel had an appointment with Dr. Koenig, a four-month follow-up from her previous visit. I parked on the second floor of the parking deck which allowed us to walk directly to Dr. Koenig's office on the second floor of the Arch Building. Muriel signed in, and as before we found a seat among the many oncology patients. I was once again struck by the unending flow of patients in some stage of their cancer treatment. It was yet another of those bittersweet moments that forced me to appreciate Muriel's progress all the more. She was eventually called by the nurse who recorded her weight (133 pounds) and blood pressure (128/82) and then assigned her to an examination room. Since Muriel had added several new prescriptions, she provided the nurse with an up-to-date list of her medications.

By the time Dr. Koenig arrived, he had reviewed the list, paying extra attention to the new prescriptions that had been prescribed by Dr. Abood. He greeted us and asked, "How are the puffers working for you?"

Muriel answered, "I'm happy to report that I've noticed a marked improvement in my breathing."

"That's great. How about your hot flashes?"

"I tried some vitamins and herbals and they seemed to help some, but since I was still having hot flashes Dr. Abood prescribed Bellergal-S."

"And has that been helpful?"

"Well, it has only been a few days since I started taking it, so I haven't noticed any difference just yet."

"Hopefully that will change, but tell Dr. Abood if it doesn't."

"I will."

Dr. Koenig nodded and then proceeded to examine Muriel. When he finished he smiled at her and said, "I see no evidence of cancer at this time, but be sure to let Dr. Abood know right away if anything of concern arises. Hopefully there will be no need for that and you can enjoy the rest of the spring without worries, but we do want to do our best to remain vigilant and stay ahead of this."

"Of course."

"The tamoxifen treatment is a component of that vigilance. I saw that Dr. Abood had considered raloxifene but since we can't prescribe them both at the same time, I recommend we stay with the tamoxifen. Unless something develops in the coming months, I'll see you for your 4-month follow-up around the end of July. Enjoy the 4th."

"You too."

We thanked him and on the way out made an appointment to return in four months. We were both relieved that Dr. Koenig had validated Muriel's positive self-assessment. Everything looks good and, more importantly, she has been feeling quite well. Part of my vigilance is to pray often and as we made our way home I offered God another prayer of thanks.

Friday, March 31, 2000

We ended the month by going out to dinner and then to a Cleveland Orchestra concert at Severance Hall. The music director, Christoph von Dohnányi, was the conductor for the evening and selected two pieces, Symphony No. 4 by Ives and the Violin Concerto by Brahms. The performance of the solo violinist, Pamela Frank, was superb, displaying her wonderful, passionate technique we both greatly appreciated.

April to mid-May 2000

This period of time was characteristic for spring in the lives of this retired couple. Muriel typically slept in while I was up each morning to do my exercises and run errands. Resuming my role as secretary, I went about setting up the Stow Senior Men's Golf League for the 2000 season. We went to Lenten services leading into Maundy Thursday, Good Friday, and ultimately the celebration of Easter. We went to concerts and dined out. As we moved into May and the weather became more consistently pleasant, I continued to put in an hour each day cleaning up our backyard.

We had moved to our present address in 1974. We were the first people to move into this development which had been literally carved out of a totally wooded area. Trees were uprooted and a street was paved right through the center. Most houses did not have any trees in the front but all the trees were left standing in the backyard. At the time we moved in we had a feral backyard that contained 42 trees of various sizes and shapes, most of which were sassafras. There was modest grading to the backside of the house but for the most part the clutch of weeds and undergrowth began about 15 feet beyond the house.

Over the years, working an hour at a time, I had managed to provide some semblance of a backyard, reclaiming a little more than half of the yard as lawn. I considered that a small victory considering the size of the task and the obstacles I faced. I cannot say for sure that it was the neighbors who lived directly behind us or prior residents of those homes, but someone had used what became our backyard as a refuse dump. That, and golf weather, served as deterrents for me to ever get the backyard completely cleaned up, so half done was an accomplishment already. But I did yearn to one day enjoy the pleasantness of a complete backyard, so for the last couple of years I was determined to finally get my backyard completely cleaned out and then to plant grass seed. I had removed about half of the trees by digging out a two-foot circle around each of them until the roots were fully exposed. Then I would cut the roots one by one until the tree came gently crashing to the ground. I was very fortunate that none of the trees hit the house. However, I did drop one tree on my neighbor's fence, wiping out a few boards but doing no significant damage.

With half the trees gone I next wanted to remove all of the debris and get the area leveled and seeded, but another obstacle in the form of poison ivy tested my resolve. The uncultivated portion of the backyard was overrun with it, and I had already had one unpleasant encounter. I had been using gloves and had my arms covered but still managed to get some exposure to the oil from the leaves. I had blotches on my arms, face, and neck that blistered and itched and eventually ran their course. Such experiences tempered my eagerness to tackle the remainder of the poison ivy.

Thursday, May 18, 2000

Today Muriel decided that she would be very helpful and assist me with the poison ivy area in the backyard. She said she was unaffected by poison ivy so I was quite happy to have her help. We still incorporated the usual precautions of using gloves and covering up our arms and legs. We worked for more than an hour and Muriel seemed to suffer no ill effects from handling the poison ivy.

As we were wrapping up our efforts for the day I said, "Maybe we can actually finally get this done. Thanks a lot for helping me out."

"I'm glad I could help, and yes, we can do this God-willing. We make a great team."

"Who, you and God?"

"Us and Him," she responded, walking over to me and offering me a quick kiss on the lips. I was convinced. We can get it done. We hadn't finished the work so we set aside our clothes to use the next day when we would hopefully complete the job.

Friday, May 19, 2000

Once again we suited up to work in the backyard. Within an hour we had pulled up and bagged the rest of the poison ivy. We then raked up and disposed of the other debris, and for another hour I carried and stacked the bags by the garage as an interim storage place. Soon they would find their way to the curb and ultimately a landfill. As I stepped back and looked upon the large pile we had amassed, I was profoundly grateful for my team.

In the late afternoon we attended the wedding of Gina d'Amico, daughter of Sue, the accompanist for the Chorale. We also attended the reception which included a sit-down dinner. We had an enjoyable time and took the opportunity to dance when there were some slow pieces, but by the time we departed Muriel began to have some itching problems. Apparently her immunity to poison ivy is not a reality and I immediately regretted having allowed her to help me in the backyard. When we got home we put Benadryl cream on those areas that had begun to blister to reduce the itching.

Sunday, May 21, 2000

This morning it was very evident that Muriel is not at all immune to poison ivy, and the regret I had felt the night before had turned to full-blown guilt. She had broken out on her face, arms, neck, back, and legs and was having a very uncomfortable time. We again applied Benadryl cream where we could to relieve the itching. I went to church and when I came home it had become obvious that more needed to be done to relieve the discomfort Muriel was experiencing from the poison ivy.

"Let me take you to one of those medical clinics," I suggested.

"Do you know where there is one?"

"I think there is one on Graham Road in Stow but let me check."

I consulted the Yellow Pages and confirmed I was correct, so we got in the car and drove the short distance to Stow. She was seen by Dr. Battles and was given a cortisone shot. In addition, he provided her with a prescription for Zyrtec. Muriel spent the rest of the day trying not to scratch all of the open blisters that resulted from the poison ivy. She was not a happy camper. I have been amazed by the great resilience she had displayed during the whole process of her cancer treatment, so it is especially difficult to witness her disappointment at now being laid low by poison ivy.

Tuesday, May 23, 2000

The visit to the clinic had provided some relief for Muriel but not at a pace sufficient to suit her, so she called Dr. Abood's office and indicated what had happened over the weekend. He agreed to call in a prescription for Medrol. Dr. Abood also indicated that should Muriel not be feeling better by Friday that she should come in to see him.

Friday, May 26, 2000

From Muriel's perspective there did not seem to be much improvement in relief from the poison ivy. Her face had improved somewhat but there seemed to be new outbreaks in other parts of her body. As a result we visited Dr. Abood's office as he had suggested on Tuesday. Dottie, Dr. Abood's nurse, took her blood pressure (120/80), temperature (98°), and pulse (76). Dr. Abood examined her very thoroughly and said, "You have some crusting and weeping, but that will not cause the poison ivy to spread. It's just a result of the blistering. I'm prescribing prednisone and hydroxyzine to help with the drying-up process and to relieve the itching. Unfortunately that's about all we can do. It'll need to run its course and I would recommend you take it easy for a few more days while that happens."

She agreed with him though I could tell by her expression that she was a bit deflated at the prospect of enduring several more days of discomfort. We thanked him and left, stopping at CVS on the way home to drop off the prescriptions which I picked up later in the day. Muriel made light of the uncomfortable situation and I joined her in the effort. We watched some videos from her collection and did a jigsaw puzzle. We read and relaxed and just enjoyed each other's company. The ordeal has actually turned out to be quite a blessing, and the guilt I had felt initially again gave way to thanks as I realized the experience was one of many that strengthened our unity over the years. When one pauses to reflect upon our experiences, the belief that we are always blessed, even when facing adversity, is overpowering.

June 2000

After a few more days the poison ivy cleared up and we returned to our more typical routines. I was left to wonder whether it was the combination of all of the medicines that had finally ended this unpleasant experience with poison ivy, or had it simply run its course. Either way, we felt fortunate to have overcome it together.

Despite such obstacles as poison ivy, overall we enjoyed the months of May and June, occasionally golfing together on Fridays and slowly chipping away further at the backyard. We spent a beautiful week at Fairfield Glade in Tennessee, where I played golf on the four resort courses while Muriel chose to spend much of her time reading. The Glade has many paved hiking trails so we walked a lot and also used the indoor swimming pool. As per our usual routine, we had prepared meals ahead of time and mostly ate in. If one desired to eat out, the choices were limited. It was either the country club restaurants or a drive to Crossville, the town closest to the resort. We did take part in the fish fry held in a very nice setting down by one of the local lakes.

We returned home for a restful end to the remainder of the first half of the year.

July to December 2000

We are enjoying what on the surface is a cancer-free lifestyle though Muriel has stayed connected with her support group by attending their monthly meetings. In addition, four of the members, including Muriel, meet once a month for a luncheon. Muriel has found great comfort from these women who have had similar experiences. I can't say enough about what the support group has meant to Muriel. One of the lasting lessons I learned from Muriel's adventure is how important it is for one to seek such support when facing some challenging circumstance. By becoming part of a group that attests to the same problem or experience one is having, one connects with that great reservoir of knowledge, comfort, and hope that so often eludes those who attempt to tackle a challenge on their own. This, obviously, is why the twelve-step program of AA has been so successful and the proof is in the results. While I realize my conclusions are no great epiphany, having witnessed firsthand the tremendous influence Muriel's support group offered her leaves me no choice but to herald the power of such groups to affect positive change in those who partake in them. I strongly believe that all persons who have or have had cancer should be encouraged to attend a support group. It would likely be good for their spouses as well. We who have not specifically experienced cancer may find it difficult to fully comprehend what the patient is actually experiencing, but associating with others who do understand provides comfort for each of us.

Muriel had a regular check-up with Dr. Abood in July and again in October. The same was true with Dr. Koenig. All seemed well and by the fall Muriel was back directing the Chorale and continuing her involvement in Stephen Ministry at church. We finally gave up our tickets for the Cleveland Orchestra but did renew our tickets to the Akron Symphony Orchestra. Thanks to Akron Metro Parks, we added another Fall Hiking Spree medallion to our walking sticks as we hiked all 13 trails.

In August we traveled to Myrtle Beach and in September we took the Rhine, Main, Danube River Cruise with Grand Circle Travel. It was a fantastic trip that began in Amsterdam then traveled down the Rhine River until we took a left onto the Main River. We traversed the Main Canal which has 66 locks that first raised, then lowered the ship as we sailed into the Danube River. We made many stops along the way enjoying the cities of Cologne, Frankfurt, Würzburg, Bamberg. Nuremberg, and ultimately, Vienna. We also enjoyed the stops at other small towns along the route and had a truly wonderful time.

In October we took a trip to Florida where we spent a week at Lehigh Acres, a resort near Fort Myers. On our return trip we visited with my two sisters, Jean and Karen, who both lived on the Gulf side about mid-state. We spent a few more days in Myrtle Beach and then continued on to Washington, D.C. before returning home. In November I booked a trip to Brechin, Ontario with the intent of doing a lot of skiing, but early on I took a nasty spill and only skied two times while we were there. It was after this last trip of the year that Muriel asked, "Are we ever going to stop traveling?"

I answered her question with a question of my own. "When you're retired, aren't you supposed to travel?"

We passed through the seasons and ended the year with a sense that bigger and brighter things are on the horizon.

< 8 >
METASTASIS I: RADIATION ROUND TWO

Saturday, January 13, 2001

We returned from Texas on the 4th, where we had spent Christmas and New Years, and just had time to unpack, wash some clothes, and repack for a trip to Bayse, Virginia. I had booked a ski week at Bryce Resort and on the 6th we were on our way. We left on I-76 and headed southeast until it merged with I-70. With three-quarters of the trip behind us, we turned south onto I-81 until we reached the exit for the resort. We had a first-floor condo, which allowed me to ski right out the front door and down to the ticket area, an awesome experience. There were five basic runs comprised primarily of man-made snow. The weather for the week was absolutely gorgeous. In the morning temperatures were below freezing, which made for good skiing conditions. By lunchtime the temperature reached the low forties and warmed up even further as the day progressed. Had I brought my golf clubs I could have golfed in the afternoon on the resort's course. Instead I was more than happy to ski each morning and go walking with Muriel in the afternoon on the roadways and trails associated with the resort.

Early in the week during one of our afternoon walks, I noticed Muriel was having difficulty lifting her left leg as she approached a curb. "What's with the gimpy leg?" I asked.

"I'm having pain in my groin area when I stride out, and it especially hurts when I step up on a curb."

"Did you pull a muscle?"

"I may have but I don't recall any specific time when I might have done that."

"Well, you'll be seeing Dr. Koenig some time after we get back, so let's make sure you tell him about this."

"I will, but hopefully it will go away before then."

We continued to walk each afternoon and I became more aware of her wincing each time she stepped up on a curb. It has been over two years since Muriel's initial diagnosis so I don't think either of us thinks the pain she is experiencing is cancer-related. If Muriel does, she does not share it with me.

With our lack of time to prepare meals prior to our departure, we had just taken recipes from Muriel's vacation file and stopped at the grocer to buy the things we would need to make our meals for the week. We both brought along books to read and I brought a puzzle as well. Despite Muriel's pain, we both had a nice relaxing week.

We returned to Munroe Falls today and in the evening we attended a 50th birthday party for Sue d'Amico. Her husband had arranged a surprise dinner party for her and about 75 guests, including her mother and sisters who had driven in from Pittsburgh to be a part of the celebration. There were gag gifts and sentimental gifts and we all had a good time.

Thursday, January 18, 2001

This morning we were once again at 95 Arch Street in Akron, the office of Dr. Koenig. And once again nearly all of the seats in the waiting room were filled. Over two years we have been coming here and always there are people waiting. Progress is surely being made with respect to surviving cancer, otherwise there wouldn't be all of these people in the offices of oncologists. It was different when I was growing up. I sometimes heard tales of individuals going to the hospital for cancer surgery only to have the doctor find that the cancer appeared to be too advanced. The person was stitched up and sent home to die, the main goal becoming pain management. Given how different Muriel's adventure has been thus far, we are very thankful for the research and progress that has been made to care for victims of cancer.

Muriel checked in and was soon called by the nurse. She was weighed (139½ pounds) and had her blood pressure taken (150/90). Muriel handed the nurse a new printout of her medications, put on the paper blouse, took a seat on the examination table, and waited for Dr. Koenig. When he entered he gave Muriel a cheery "Hello, how are you doing?" as he crossed the room to wash his hands.

"Not so good. I'm having an intermittent pain in my shoulder which makes it difficult to raise my arm, and a pretty persistent pain in the groin area which hurts when I walk, especially if I raise my leg to step up. I think I might have pulled a muscle in the groin area."

Muriel's revelation about the pain in the shoulder was news to me.

Dr. Koenig said, "I'm sorry to hear that. When did you first have the pain?"

"I've had the pain in the groin for maybe two, three weeks, but the pain in the shoulder is new in the last few days."

"Ibuprofen will be good for pain relief and before you leave I'll give you some samples of Vioxx." An examination of Muriel followed and when he was done, he said, "I don't think it is a metastasis of the breast cancer, but we can't be sure without further information. I would like you to have a bone scan and a CT scan of the chest, abdomen, and pelvic area. We'll compare those scans to the initial base scans. I'll see you back in one month so we can discuss the results."

In Dr. Koenig's opinion metastasis appeared not to be a factor, but having the tests will provide a definitive answer. Before leaving the office I made all of the appointments for the different scans requested by Dr. Koenig. Fortunately the tests were scheduled for the same day, January 30th. How's that for an anniversary present? We had little conversation in the car and when I got her home she encouraged me to go and play bridge at church. She said, "There is nothing we can do until we see the results of the scans." So I took her advice and went to play bridge.

Friday, January 19, 2001

The new Chorale season is about to begin and Muriel wants to be prepared. She had listened to CDs that publishers had sent her and has selected several new pieces. The music she had ordered had arrived and our goal for the day was to assemble the music into folders for each of the singers. The sheets were three-hole punched and then collated for insertion into a plastic binder. In keeping with Muriel's organizational skills, each piece of music was numbered and each folder was assembled with pieces of music all bearing the same number. I was in charge of punching and collating, and, having accomplished this task before lunchtime, I went skiing in the afternoon with Muriel's blessing.

Tuesday, January 30, 2001

We wished each other a happy anniversary, number 42, and shared the common anniversary card, but after that we drove to City Hospital where Muriel was scheduled to have a bone scan at 7:00 and a CT scan at 8:00 that was to cover the chest, abdomen, and pelvic area. The bone scan was routine, but the CT scan turned out to be very difficult for Muriel when the technician attempted to start an IV. Since there was no longer a port available, it was necessary to utilize a vein in the arm. However, that vein turned out to be uncooperative and an attempt was made to access a vein in the wrist. That too proved painfully futile, and to reduce the trauma Muriel was experiencing we were left alone, giving Muriel the opportunity to recover before the test was begun.

After Muriel calmed down I left the examination area. The test proceeded without an IV and no contrast was able to be made. When the scan was over I put my arm around her and walked her to the car, making sure we encountered no curbs or stairs along the way. We knew Muriel was having pain in the area where the leg joins the hip, but we needed to wait until we saw Dr. Koenig before we knew exactly what the scans had determined.

It may have been one of the first times on our anniversary that we did not have our usual Duckling Rosé dinner. After Muriel's ordeal with the CT scan I judged it best that she relax for the rest of the day. I ended up cutting up veggies and we had a chicken stir fry with rice. It went well with the rosé wine we had gotten for the duckling. We are one year closer to the magic fifty.

Wednesday, January 31, 2001

It would be a stretch to think that Muriel was thinking about her death, but today we packed up all of her jewelry and took it in to C. L. Davis to have it appraised. There had been times that she had mentioned that she would like to pass all of her jewelry on to her daughter, granddaughters, and daughter-in-law. We also made the journey to Canton to meet with our accountant and talk about our income tax. After we returned home I made some bread in the bread maker Muriel had gotten me for Christmas.

Friday, February 2, 2001

This evening we went out to dinner at Applebee's and then to E. J. Thomas Hall where we again attended the ballet, another of the arts Muriel had introduced to me. Living in Fort Lee, New Jersey she had often attended the New York City Ballet with her father and saw the likes of Jacque d'Amboise and Maria Tallchief. Ohio Ballet, under the direction of Heinz Poll, is an above-average resident company that often travels to other parts of the country to display their abilities. At Muriel's insistence we had been season ticket holders for several years, enjoying the three performances that were given each season.

Saturday, February 10, 2001

On the morning of February 3rd, we had the car packed early and left once again for Bayse, Virginia where I had lined up another week of skiing and relaxing at Bryce Resort. I skied every morning and we took walks in the afternoon. This time though we made sure that the paths we took did not cause Muriel to have to step up onto a curb, causing her undue pain. Even though Muriel had had the two scans, we were still in the dark as to the nature of the problem. In addition to the ibuprofen, the use of Vioxx provided further relief when a higher level of pain was present. I had brought a 1000-piece jigsaw puzzle plus a couple of books and Muriel had brought her usual complement of seven books. We had prepared meals ahead of time and I did all of the cooking and clean-up. It was another nice, quiet week.

We returned from Virginia today, arriving home in midafternoon. We unpacked, freshened up, and then went to Applebee's for dinner. I ordered the basket of ribs with fries and a tall Killian's Red. Muriel had the petite steak with grilled vegetables and a glass of Merlot. Since we pretty much adhere to a regimen of chicken, fish, and turkey at home, we tend to drop all rules when we dine out.

Ever since our first ski trip to Virginia and the first sign of pain in Muriel's groin, there seems to be an elephant in the room that no one is talking about. I certainly do not want to speculate that the cancer has returned, and I'm sure that Muriel doesn't want to think about that either. So our conversation skirted the subject except to discuss the fact that she has an appointment with Dr. Koenig later in the week.

We completed the evening by going to the concert given by the Akron Symphony Orchestra. Ya-Hui Wang, the new music director of the orchestra, was the conductor for the evening and had selected three pieces for our enjoyment. The first was Antonín Dvořák's Symphony No. 8 in G Major, Op. 88, B.163. Composed in 1889 and premiered the following year in Prague, it did not have the pizzazz of his more famous Ninth Symphony, *From the New World*, but was very melodic and set the stage nicely for the second piece prior to intermission, "Winter" from *The Seasons* by Glazunov. The second half of the program featured

Cho-Liang Lin on the solo violin playing the Concerto for Violin and Orchestra in D Major, Op. 50 by Tyzen Hsiao. There was a certain warmth throughout the program's entirety and we all went home pleased with our new music director and the music she had selected.

Monday, February 12, 2001

Muriel was up bright and early this morning because today is the day we were to find out about the scans she had undergone on January 30th. However, before we went to Dr. Koenig's office Muriel was scheduled to see Dr. Karlen, her oncological gynecologist, for an examination and Pap smear. We then came down two floors in the Arch Street building to Dr. Koenig's office. We sat for a few minutes before Muriel was called into the examination area by Beth. She was weighed (139½ pounds) and had her blood pressure taken (140/90). Muriel provided the nurse with an update on the medications that she was taking, and we were left to wait for Dr. Koenig. Muriel sat on the examination table and I was seated on a chair halfway across the room from her. With a palpable anxiousness present, we waited.

Dr. Koenig arrived with a large envelope that presumably contained the scan results and greeted us as he crossed to the sink to wash his hands. He seemed subdued, though I suspect that having to tell a patient that the cancer has spread is never a pleasant task. One certainly cannot anticipate how the patient is going to react. Nevertheless he withdrew the scans from the envelope and placed them on a fluorescent screen and switched it on. He began to speak immediately. "When we compare these scans with the base scans we can see significant changes." He pointed with his finger and continued, "Each of the white spots you see on the bones represents a cancerous tumor that we'll need to deal with. There also seems to be a lesion on your liver, but we can't be sure because of the lack of contrast when the scans were made."

Muriel could no longer remain silent. "What does all that mean?"

"Unfortunately Muriel, the breast cancer has metastasized to the bone and, it appears, to your liver."

Muriel and I both looked to the floor, quietly trying to digest the bad news for a moment. It was what we had each privately worried might be, but having that worry come to realization shocks and saddens in an instant. I was reeling. The elephant in the room was now standing in full view. It was difficult for me to gauge how Muriel was taking this news, but I was certainly quite shaken. I only drew my gaze up from the floor when I heard Muriel ask, "Where do we go from here?"

113

Dr. Koenig answered, "I recommend that you have radiation therapy again to shrink and kill the tumors in the bone, and possibly later on have some additional chemotherapy."

"Will further treatment curtail the spread of the cancer?"

"I can't guarantee that."

Dr. Koenig explained that the usual places of metastasis are bone, brain, liver, and lungs. Muriel had two of the four and could very likely have the other two somewhere down the road. He added, "Muriel, cancer is a metastatic disease, and in a case such as yours, it's incurable."

I still could not gauge Muriel's reaction, but I was devastated within. I searched for peace, but at that moment I only found pain. My beautiful wife of 42 years, mother of my two wonderful children and Oma to four more, had just been told that she would die from her cancer. I had solemnly accepted news of her original diagnosis as she had been the one who had gently told me. Hearing an even worse diagnosis from a third party, albeit gently as well, was proving to be too much for me to bear. I felt like screaming away some of the pain, but restraint and shock saved me from upsetting us further. Muriel finally broke the silence.

"I want to have whatever treatment is available that will help me to prolong my life."

"Of course. We will provide those treatments for you."

They discussed the doctor's proposed course of action and she was given a physical examination. The shock had dissipated a bit but the pain had not. I said little. Dr. Koenig asked her to stop taking tamoxifen and gave her a new prescription for Arimidex, as well as hydrocodone for pain relief. We left the examination area, but before leaving the office I made an appointment with the radiation therapy department for Thursday.

I gripped Muriel's hand and we slowly walked back toward the car. I suggested we go out for lunch and she mumbled an acceptance to my offer. It was now clear that she too was shaken. It was a short drive to the Rockne's restaurant at Barney's Corners. We asked for a booth and I ordered a tall Killian's Red for me and a Scotch on the rocks for Muriel. She still had not said anything. When our drinks arrived I quietly said, "I'm sorry sweetheart." The first word out of Muriel was singular in nature and expressed it all. "Shit!"

We sat for a few moments with hands clasped across the table as tears began to stream down our cheeks. I think we both knew that at this point it was just a matter of time before Muriel would die. In the midst of our streaming tears Muriel said, "The adventure goes on. It's just on a different track."

I nodded as she continued. "Please promise me that you will do all within your power to ensure that I will not experience undue pain as this adventure continues."

"I promise."

The main thrust of the remainder of our conversation concerned minimizing her pain and going as far as we can together. We had just celebrated our 42nd wedding anniversary and Muriel had set a goal of making it to our 50th. I came to the realization that this goal will probably not be achieved, but I am determined to do everything I can to prolong the time we will have left to share. We are ready to move forward, but with a slightly revised schedule. I moved to her side of the booth and gave her a big hug and a kiss. We sat side-by-side as we each enjoyed a Rueben sandwich and a heap of fries. On our way home I dropped off the prescription for Arimidex and the pain killer Dr. Koenig had prescribed, which I picked up later in the day. With the big lunch we didn't worry about dinner and spent the evening cuddled on the couch watching one of Muriel's "feel good" movies.

Thursday, February 15, 2001

This morning we were up early in preparation for an appointment at 10:00 in the radiation therapy department of City Hospital. The mood was less solemn, but remained subdued as we each came to grips with the new direction Muriel's adventure would be taking. Still, I gained strength as I watched Muriel continue her rebound and again allow herself God's peace. We were in the waiting room by ten to the hour and just like the oncologist's office, there were persons garbed in hospital gowns awaiting radiation treatment. We were ushered into an examination room followed immediately by our favorite radiation oncologist, Dr. Doncals. She greeted us like friends she had not seen in some time, immediately putting us at ease.

She briefly reviewed the results of the two scans and then shared her assessment and proposal for Muriel's treatment. "If you do as I suggest, you'll be receiving radiation to the pelvic area to relieve the pain you are experiencing and to shrink the tumors. But you need to be aware that since you've already had radiation therapy, short- and long-term difficulties may arise. You see, your body can absorb only so much radiation in a particular area. There is a mild overlap between the area of the previous dosage and the new area of radiation therapy.

Short term, you may experience fatigue and nausea, which will go away when the radiation is stopped. Long term, because of the location of the radiation in the pelvic area, you may experience some damage to the bowels which may cause diarrhea. As far as the proximity of the two treatment areas, I'm confident that there'll be no breakdown of the regular tissue in the overlapping areas. I'll give you and Keith a few minutes to discuss whether or not you wish to proceed with the radiation therapy."

Dr. Doncals left and Muriel immediately said, "What's to discuss?"

"It's your decision sweetheart, but what about the side effects?"

"I'm not really concerned about the side effects. I just want to get rid of the pain."

"Then I suppose the decision is made."

We called Dr. Doncals back in. She asked, "Would you like to proceed with the radiation?"

Muriel responded without hesitation with the exact plea she had just shared with me. "Absolutely. I just want to get rid of the pain."

"We will do our best to make you comfortable," Dr. Doncals replied. "Since you are willing to proceed you are eligible to participate in a study that will randomize you to one of two groups for the administration of the radiation treatments. I can explain the study in more detail if you think you might possibly wish to participate."

"Yes, please do."

"There will be two groups receiving radiation treatment. One group will receive a daily treatment with the typical dosage of radiation for 30 days just as you had before, while the other group will receive ten treatments over a 10-day period with three times the typical dosage. The study includes the completion of questionnaires before, during, and after the radiation. There are questions regarding your pain and the relief of that pain. It also asks questions to find out how much the treatment affects your quality of life, and how the treatment affects other aspects of your life. To participate, both you and Keith must sign an agreement to be a part of the study."

Muriel opted to participate. Dr. Doncals presented the papers and we both signed. The last item of business was a thorough examination of Muriel including a test of her strength as Dr. Doncals pushed against various extremities. When the examination was complete Muriel said, "We're scheduled to go to Texas at the beginning of March. Can the radiation therapy be postponed until we return?"

"Yes, that's no problem. I have an update on your participation in the study. You have been assigned to the group that will receive ten radiation treatments at three times the dosage you had previously received. Do you wish to continue?"

"Yes."

"All right then. Before you leave today we'll schedule your first treatment to take place soon after you return from Texas. I'm also giving you a prescription for Kadian which will help to relieve your pain."

We thanked her and made our way to the front desk. Muriel's consultation with the radiation oncologist and technician was scheduled for March 19th, four days after our expected return.

Wednesday, February 28, 2001

For the rest of the month we reverted to a mode of living indicative of Muriel's survival demeanor under God's peace, which was always present so long as we connected with it. After the initial shock we had both felt learning that the cancer had metastasized, Muriel had reverted to her usual upbeat self, embracing the mantra "this too shall pass." Fortunately and gratefully, I too feel the influence of God's peace, making the next leg of the adventure far more endurable for us both.

Thursday, March 15, 2001

On the morning of March 1st, we left for Texas to see our children and grandchildren. We had booked a one-night stay at the Fairfield Resort in Branson, Missouri. It is a beautiful place, but we were solely concerned with finding a place to rest. We continued on to Texas in the morning. We had reservations at the Comfort Inn in Plano and used that as our base of operations. On Friday we visited Muriel's sister, Judith, and her husband Richard. Judith was going to dialysis twice a week so we visited on a day when she was home. There did not seem to be any heaviness in the air despite the fact that it might be the last time Judith would see Muriel alive. We had a great visit and had dinner at a Mexican restaurant and lived it up a bit by ordering a pitcher of margaritas. It was nearly midnight when we returned to the motel.

On Saturday we stopped to visit with Kay, Larry, and our grandchildren. We spent part of the evening playing poker just for fun. Kenton kept trying to bluff us time and time again in an effort to win the pot. On Sunday we went to Mark's house bright and early to pick up Meagan to take her to Angel Fire, New Mexico where we had booked a cabin for the week. I planned on taking Meagan skiing for her first time. We drove the 600-plus miles all in one day and Meagan was very helpful in getting the car unloaded. Muriel took the downstairs bedroom while Meagan took the bedroom upstairs and I bunked in the loft area. That way we were all able to do our own thing and not disturb each other.

The next morning, Meagan and I went to rent her some skis and I signed her up for lessons on Tuesday. She took a lesson in the morning and another in the afternoon and then she and I skied together. Angel Fire was the place I had learned to ski and there is one trail, a green (beginner), that is 3½ miles long running down the backside of the mountain. It was a wonderful trail for the two of us to ski together and we had great fun, so much so that we went skiing two other days. Muriel had brought her books and we also had a 1000-piece jigsaw puzzle which I, with Meagan's help, assembled during the week. One morning there was fresh snow so we built a snowman.

The last night we went out to dinner at a restaurant right near the quad lift. Just before we were to be served our food, the electricity failed. Fortunately for us our orders were ready and we ate by candlelight at our table. When we returned to the cabin we decided to pack up and leave for Texas. We had been informed that the electrical grid was down in the northeast corner of New Mexico and there was no prospect of restoring electricity for the rest of the night. So with a couple of candles and two flashlights, we managed to get everything packed up and into the car. Meagan was a terrific helper and she insisted that Muriel do nothing except relax until we had everything loaded. We were underway by 9:00 and had driven about 12 miles when we discovered that the whole northeast electrical grid was not down. Nonetheless, we decided to continue on and stopped at a Best Western at around two in the morning. We had no problem falling asleep. We had breakfast at the motel and continued on to Texas to spend a little more time with family before returning to Ohio on the 15th.

Monday, March 19, 2001

This morning Muriel had an appointment in the radiation therapy department to have the radiation oncologist and the technician determine exactly where on her body she would receive the radiation therapy treatment. The business was completed in good order and we were back home within the hour.

Wednesday, March 21, 2001

Yesterday morning I took Muriel to the radiation therapy department, as it was necessary to have what is called, in their parlance, a radiation simulation. This morning we returned for Muriel's first session. Muriel is still suffering from the pain in her pelvic area, though her use of Kadian has helped to minimize the pain. Her spirits are good and she is ready to have the ten rounds of radiation therapy.

Friday, March 23, 2001

Today was the second session of radiation therapy. We have already adapted back to our previous routine. I drop Muriel at the door and park the car while she walks through to the radiation therapy department, dons a hospital gown, and takes a seat to wait to be called in for her treatment. I get the parking pass stamped and join her, prepared to hold her pocketbook when she goes in for her treatment. As part of the Radiation Therapy Oncology Group study Muriel is participating in, today was a quality assurance day so she spoke with the administrator of the group study and completed a questionnaire.

In the evening we went out to dinner and then to E. J. Thomas Hall where we were entertained by Harvey Korman and Tim Conway. One of the great by-products of watching the two of them doing skits is the way they crack each other up. It was a wonderfully humorous show and it came at a great time. I judge we both need to have a few more laughs in our lives.

Monday, March 26, 2001

Today was radiation therapy treatment number three. Prior to the therapy we met with Dr. Doncals, who physically examined Muriel. She then asked, "Have the initial treatments had any effect on the pain you are experiencing?"

"There has been very little relief thus far, though I suppose that's to be expected given I've had just two treatments."

"I'm optimistic that will change as you undergo more treatments. In the meantime continue to use the Kadian to help control the pain."

From radiation therapy we took the elevator to the second floor, crossed the bridge from the hospital to the physician's office building, and entered Dr. Koenig's office where Muriel had an appointment.

After the nurse did a check of her vital signs, Dr. Koenig entered and performed a physical examination. He then sat down on his stool and said, "I want to give you some information about Aredia. It is a bone reabsorption inhibitor administered intravenously for the treatment of osteolytic bone metastases of breast cancer. In simpler terms, the breast cancer metastasizes causing tumors in the bone, which in turn would leave holes in the bone when radiation kills the tumors. So to ensure that the bone is not weakened further, making it subject to fracture, it's necessary to fill in the holes. Aredia is a biphosphate that adheres to the bone and essentially becomes the filler in the holes. I urge you to be a part of this therapy, but there are side effects and of course it is your decision to make."

Without hesitation Muriel said, "Of course I want to do this, but I would like to learn more about the potential side effects."

"I have some literature for you which lists all of the different side effects. Twelve of those qualify as severe." With that note my ears perked up. He continued, "But in clinical trials, individual patients mostly experienced individual side effects, and some had none at all."

"That sounds better than a fractured pelvis or broken hip," Muriel said with a grin.

"Yes, that is why I'm recommending it. A fracture is the last thing you need right now. If you review the literature and still want to proceed, we can begin Aredia treatments today."

"Don't I have to be done with the radiation before we begin?"

"No, the radiation is already killing the tumors and we want to get right to work on filling the holes in the bone. We would do this once a month and I want you to record any side effects you may experience so we can discuss them at your next appointment. Give this material a read and talk about it. I'll be back in a little bit to see what you think."

"That's all right," Muriel interjected. "Let's just move forward with the treatment."

"Very well," Dr. Koenig replied.

The word "severe" had certainly caught my attention, but if Muriel was willing to proceed, I was not going to dissuade her. We filed from the examination room to the treatment room where Muriel took up her usual place in the chair in the back corner of the room. We were fortunate to have one of Dr. Koenig's most adept nurses, Beth Stein, set up the IV. She just seemed to have the perfect technique to find a vein without causing Muriel undue discomfort. Initially blood was drawn and then the Aredia treatment began. The 90 mg drip was regulated for completion in 90 minutes. I sat on a stool next to Muriel's chair and we both read as patients shuttled in and out for chemotherapy treatments. The nursing staff maintained a sense of order in the chaos of activity. Laughter and conversation filled the room as another day played out in Muriel's adventure. We returned home and had soup for lunch. Then Muriel made a bowl of popcorn, grabbed the current book she was reading, and climbed into the waterbed for the rest of the day. I guess she figured she had had enough excitement for one day.

Wednesday, March 28, 2001

Yesterday we had gotten a call from Dr. Koenig's office explaining there had been a problem with Muriel's blood test on Monday, so in addition to radiation therapy treatment today, it was necessary to go back to Dr. Koenig's office so Muriel could have another blood draw. I held her hand as the hematology technician searched for a usable vein. With the prospect of monthly Aredia treatments Muriel rues the day she had the port removed, but she also is not interested in having a new port put in place. The blood draw was completed without further mishap and we drove back to our house. Even though April is just around the corner, there seems to be a chill in the air. I made a fire in the fireplace so Muriel could watch a movie in comfort while I cleaned up in the basement.

Friday, March 30, 2001

For the fifth time this week we were at the radiation therapy department, on this occasion for Muriel's seventh overall treatment. Today was also a follow-up day for her participation in the study and she thus had to complete a questionnaire again. After therapy we went to Giant Eagle to do the monthly shopping. Muriel had been busy preparing her menus during the week and had completed her shopping list and clipped her coupons, so we were our usual efficient selves: up one aisle, down the next, etc., and finally to the cashier and out the door.

Saturday, March 31, 2001

It is the last day of the month and we do not have to go to radiation therapy. With 70 percent of the radiation complete Muriel is beginning to feel a lessening of the pain. She still has used the pain medicine as she feels a need, but has tapered off significantly. I washed sheets and made the beds and in the evening we went out to dinner at Applebee's on the way to E. J. Thomas Hall. Muriel has recovered well from her "setback" and is her old optimistic self again. Ya-Hui Wang once again conducted the Akron Symphony Orchestra and for tonight's concert she had selected a very eclectic program. It began with Samuel Barber's *Adagio for Strings*. We sat mesmerized through the whole work as the music soared through the sonorities of the piece. It is just one of those arrangements that, as we held hands, drew us closer together as we shared in its beauty. The second piece was "The Promise of Living" from *The Tender Land* by Aaron Copland. In addition to the music, we were further immersed in the presentation through the wonderful photochoreography of James Westwater. A large screen had been put in place above the orchestra and pictures were projected in keeping with the music. So not only did we have spectacular music, but beautiful pictures that seamlessly dissolved from one to the next, a symbiosis of sight and sound to which we were made witness. We were next treated to the Akron Symphony Chorus singing Francis Poulenc's *Gloria*. Janice Chandler was the guest soprano. The last piece for the evening was Symphony No. 3, *Rhenish*, in E-flat Major, Op. 97 by Robert Schumann. It was a fitting way to end the evening, and I know for sure this couple went home somewhat euphoric from the bombardment to our senses that this evening had delivered us.

Monday, April 2, 2001

Today is the antepenultimate day of radiation therapy and Muriel would appreciate my naming it that way. She just loved the use of words and she was so well read with a vocabulary that far exceeds mine. There were more than a couple of times that I scurried for the unabridged Oxford English Dictionary that we kept on a stand in our dining room to check out a word she had used.

All of the years we were married I had always been the one to do the crossword puzzle in the daily newspaper as well as the *New York Times* puzzle on Sunday. It wasn't until her cancer had reappeared that she shared with me that she too liked to do crossword puzzles. So from then on I bought her a crossword puzzle book each month, and there were many times when she would return from radiation therapy or an Aredia treatment and spend the rest of the day working on crossword puzzles. She liked the books where the puzzles were graded easy, medium, hard, and difficult. She rarely did all of the puzzles in one section before moving on but would move from section to section as she felt challenged that day. Considering her penchant for perfection I fully expected that she would add another book to our library, that being the *New York Times Crossword Puzzle Dictionary*. However, she never did, and if she were stumped on any given day she would check the answers in the back to get back on track.

Since it was Monday we were scheduled to see Dr. Doncals after her radiation therapy treatment. Visiting with Dr. Doncals is always an uplifting experience. She is always so positive and extremely thorough, and we both feel fortunate to have her as Muriel's radiation oncologist. She put Muriel through the usual physical resistance tests and gave her a thorough physical examination. Muriel shared feedback with Dr. Doncals, letting her know that there has been significant reduction in the groin-area pain and that she has been taking less pain medication.

Tuesday, April 3, 2001

Today was another doubleheader day. We began the morning with radiation therapy and after lunch had an appointment with Dr. Abood in Kent. Dottie took her vital signs: blood pressure (115/70), weight (138 pounds), pulse (80), and then a new data point was added to assess the level of pain Muriel was experiencing on a scale of zero to ten (five). Muriel brought Dr. Abood up to date on all that had happened since her last visit in February. He asked about the medications she was taking and whether or not she was having any complications. She explained the difficulty of being plagued both ways with respect to her bowel movements. She was taking Senocot for constipation, but two to three days later she would take Kadian to shut down her diarrhea. He thought that some of the difficulty was due to the radiation treatments she is presently getting and let her know that if the problems persist after she completed her cycle, he would investigate further. Muriel spoke of having bicep pain and shoulder discomfort, particularly as it pertained to scratching or washing her back. Dr. Abood suggested some exercises to help loosen up her shoulder and indicated that she might also want to try Celebrex, an anti-inflammatory drug. Before we left Muriel scheduled a follow-up appointment in August.

< 9 >
AREDIA AND RADIATION AFTERMATH

Thursday, April 5, 2001

Muriel had completed her radiation therapy yesterday, but was feeling rather under the weather today. She awoke at 11:00, took her medications, had a piece of toast, and went back to bed. I checked on her before I went off to play bridge at church. She was reading.

"Are you feeling any better?"

"I'm still feeling a little nauseous."

"Should I stay home in case it gets worse?"

"No, I'll be okay. You go and play bridge."

I accepted her assurances and kissed her goodbye. "I love you. Call if you need me."

I had probably been playing bridge for a half hour when Rita, the office secretary, came into the room and said, "Muriel called. She would like you to come home."

I departed without hesitation and now encountered the same nine traffic lights in reverse order as I hurried from church to home. When I finally arrived, I moved quickly upstairs and found Muriel still in bed. "Are you all right?"

"I threw up and had some diarrhea, but the pains across my abdomen have gotten really bad."

"I'll call Dr. Koenig's office and see what he has to say."

I was connected to the office but their protocol was to take your name and number and call you back. I then called the radiation therapy department and asked to speak to Dr. Doncals. We were connected and I explained the situation to her. She said, "Take her to the emergency room." I helped Muriel get dressed and then we drove to Akron City Hospital. I parked in the ER parking lot and got a wheelchair for Muriel. I moved her into the ER and up to the desk where we signed in and had our medical cards checked. There was a quick triage with Muriel supplying answers to the nurse, in between pangs of pain. We were soon moved into an examination area and waited for a doctor to examine her. The ER nurse came in and took the usual vital signs. While she was completing this task Dr. Peter Listerman came into the cubicle and asked, "What brings you to emergency today?"

"I had breast cancer that metastasized to the bone and I completed radiation therapy yesterday. Later in the afternoon I began to have slight pains across my abdomen. I did manage to sleep through the night, but this morning the pain has increased. I have also had the dry heaves and some vomiting as well as diarrhea."

"Have you taken any medication for the pain?"

"Dr. Doncals had prescribed Kadian which I had been using to curtail my diarrhea and reduce the pain I had experienced prior to radiation, so I took two pills midmorning."

"Did the medication help?"

"Yes, but I don't want to just load up on meds without knowing what is causing the pain."

He did a thorough examination of Muriel, listening with his stethoscope and probing with his hands. When he was done he said, "I think we need to do some tests to help me figure out what is causing the pain and discomfort you are experiencing. First the nurse is going to hook you up to an IV so we can get some fluids back into your system."

Blood was drawn and other tests were performed. About two hours into our stay, Dr. Bender, Dr. Flynn's partner, the surgeon for Muriel's mastectomies, came to visit, and she probed and questioned Muriel. Dr. Bender said, "There is concern that you may have a bowel obstruction and that it might be necessary to have surgery."

I asked, "When will you know?"

"We'll let you know as quickly as we can."

After two more anticipatory hours in the ER, Dr. Listerman returned. "All of the tests you had were pretty much normal. However, there appeared to be little passage of air in your bowel which pointed us in the direction of a bowel obstruction. That is why Dr. Bender came in to talk to you. I also spoke with Dr. Abood and Dr. Koenig and our final conclusion is you are suffering from radiation enteritis. You will be admitted to the hospital and placed under Dr. Koenig's care in the oncology ward."

"Thank you," I said, but the tension that had built up during our wait for further word had not dissipated. I continued, "It concerns me that you have made all of these consultations with Muriel's doctors and we know nothing about it until now. There ought to be some protocols that would require a periodic check back to keep the patient informed. We have been here for four hours with no report of what is happening except for the time Dr. Bender was here."

"You, of course, are right and we need to do a better job of that. However, you need to remember that your wife is not the only patient in the emergency room."

"I do understand that, but she is the only wife I have and I need to know what is happening."

I accompanied Muriel to the oncology floor and waited while she put on her hospital gown and got comfortable in bed. She was pretty beat at this point and looked as if she would like to nap. I made arrangements to have her TV turned on, got instructions as to what she wanted me to bring in on Friday, gave her a kiss goodbye, and said, "I love you. I'll see you after lunch tomorrow. I have an appointment with my cardiologist in the morning."

"I just remembered, please call Sue Wells to tell her I can't make the support group session on Saturday, and call Sue d'Amico and tell her I won't be there to direct the Chorale on Sunday."

"I'll take care of it sweetheart."

Friday, April 6, 2001

I spent the morning calling all of those persons that needed to be informed that Muriel was in the hospital. The first call was to the church asking that Muriel be put on the prayer list. I also requested that either of the pastors visit Muriel in the hospital this afternoon so we could have Communion together. I called both of our children as well as Sue d'Amico. I next called Lois Jenkins, Muriel's Stephen minister. She said she would probably visit Muriel this evening. Sue Wells was next. She indicated she would inform the others in the support group and encourage them to visit Muriel if they were free. My appointment with Dr. Hughes was at 10:15, but he got tied up with an emergency patient and I didn't get to see him until just before noon. Needless to say my blood pressure was a little higher than expected. If the office personnel would just inform patients there would be no need to get exasperated. Two days in a row. Ugh.

I had anticipated driving home before going to the hospital to see Muriel, but the delay changed my plans. However, I had taken the precaution to bring the items that Muriel had requested yesterday. So I ate lunch in the hospital cafeteria and then went up to the 7th floor to see Muriel. She was looking much better than she had when I brought her in yesterday. "Hi sweetheart, you're looking great." I crossed to the bed and gave her a hug and a kiss.

"Thanks, I feel much better."

"Has Dr. Koenig been in to see you?"

"Yes, he was in this morning. He confirmed the diagnosis of radiation enteritis and prescribed an antibiotic, and Lomotil to calm down my stomach. The antibiotic is being given intravenously and that's why I am still hooked up."

"What have you been eating?"

"He put me on a pretty bland diet, but considering how my stomach has been feeling, that's fine with me."

Shortly after I arrived, Pastor Johnson came by. He administered Communion and then said prayers for Muriel's continued healing. I had also brought in the Phase 10 cards, which had not been on Muriel's list, so we spent some of the time playing a game. I stayed with Muriel until her dinner arrived and then departed for home.

Monday, April 9, 2001

I visited Muriel in the hospital both Saturday and Sunday, and today I went to the hospital to bring her home. I had brought clothing that she had requested the night before, and when I entered her room I was happy to see how great she looked. "How are you feeling today?"

"Much, much better and I'm eager to get back home. Dr. Koenig was in this morning as well as Dr. Doncals from radiation therapy."

"That must have been a surprise. What did she have to say?"

"She said since you had called she just wanted to check up on me, particularly whether my bone pain had diminished."

"How nice of her to stop by."

Dr. Stephens discharged Muriel into my care and provided us with two prescriptions. One was for Phenergan suppositories (25 mg) for nausea, and the other was for Lomotil for her diarrhea. A volunteer arrived with a wheelchair to take Muriel to the parking deck where I picked her up. I dropped off the two prescriptions at CVS on the way home and then got Muriel comfortable in the family room. She said she wasn't hungry, so I didn't push the matter. I called both of our children to let them know that mom is back home. I also called the church to let them know Muriel had returned from the hospital and I requested prayers of thanksgiving for next Sunday's service. Muriel was content to read and do puzzles in her crossword puzzle book.

Thursday, April 19, 2001

Since coming home from the hospital, Muriel has gradually increased the amount and types of food she is eating and has also been doing things around the house. She has gone to two Chorale practices and again provided the spark and leadership we are used to getting from her. We have a single mother of three in our church who cuts hair out of her home. Muriel wanted to try her services so I drove Muriel to her home. She was happy with the results so I guess I have lost my haircutting job. I am not unhappy about that, as it was always a little tense for fear I would hack off too much in one location and create a lopsided look.

This morning we have an appointment to see Dr. Doncals for Muriel's two-week follow-up. Rather than drop Muriel off today, she walked with me from the parking deck. We even walked outside and across the street as the much anticipated warm weather of spring was teasing us. We walked through to the radiation therapy department, had our parking ticket stamped, and were immediately directed to Dr. Doncals examination room. She greeted Muriel as she came through the door. "How are you feeling?"

"I'm happy to report that I have no pain and I have not taken any pain pills in the last four days."

"That's great. Is the diarrhea gone?"

"I haven't had a bout in three or four days, but I would like a refill of the Kadian in case I need it."

Muriel positioned herself on the examination table and Dr. Doncals proceeded with a thorough physical examination. She ran her through the usual strength routines and listened to all of her working parts with her stethoscope. "It looks like you have good movement in your legs and pelvic area," Dr. Doncals said. "Let us know if you have any reoccurring pain."

"I definitely will do that," replied Muriel. "I'll see you in two weeks."

We departed with a prescription for Kadian, with three refills. It provides Muriel with a safety net should her diarrhea return. After we arrived home we had an appointment with a plumber. As far as being a handyman, I have five thumbs on each hand so it is best that when things need fixing I call on the persons who can do the job. This may be hard to believe, but I was having the plumber investigate a leak we've had since we moved into our house in 1974. We have been thinking of selling our house and decided to address some of these kinds of things to make our home more presentable for sale. The leak had never seemed significant enough to have it taken care of earlier. It was somewhere in the upstairs bathroom and water trickled down the drainpipe and occasionally caused a small pool on the floor. Oftentimes the water would evaporate before we would even see it. As it turned out there was a nail driven into the drainpipe when the wall board was put up, so the only time there was a chance for water to leak was when we flushed the toilet or used the shower or sink. Such intermittent flows down the pipe meant that the leak was almost undetectable. In the afternoon we also had someone in from Theil's, a local cabinet restyler, who was taking all of the measurements to redo our kitchen cabinets.

It has been over a quarter century since we moved into this house. Prior to our move we had lived one street over, and while this house was being built Kay and I would walk over and follow the progress of its completion. Muriel and Mark were content to wait until we moved in. The house is a four-bedroom colonial with a full basement. There is a huge family room with a fireplace, a combined living/dining room, a full bathroom upstairs, and a half bathroom downstairs. There is also a two-car garage and a nice front porch. On the trips that Kay and I made to the house, she picked out the bedroom she wanted and when we moved in that was the one she got. Her brother was very accommodating. The fourth bedroom was turned into an office and computer room, and we later added a deck off the family room. It was all very comfortable for us but being empty nesters at this point, it seems to be a little more house than we need. I did convince Muriel to look at the new condominiums that are being constructed on the old "Baker's Acres" golf course. I think they are great and would move in a heartbeat, but she is happy with where we are.

Monday, April 23, 2001

Muriel had an appointment with Dr. Koenig, and following that, an Aredia treatment. Once again the office was nearly filled to capacity when we signed in. Apparently the game remains the same, only the players change. It is difficult to imagine that it has been nearly three years since we first began coming here. One has to just remove those kinds of thoughts from the mind, because each day is a blessing and we get to spend it together. Muriel's "Peace from God" continues to rub off on me and we continue to do what we have to do. Eventually Muriel was called into the office, weighed (134½ pounds), had her blood pressure taken (136/80), and was handed a paper blouse and asked to strip to the waist. This, of course, was not the first time for this routine. It has always been done in preparation for the doctor's examination. Dr. Koenig commented on how good she looks after her hospitalization. He examined her and we crossed the hall for her Aredia treatment.

The first chair inside the room was available so Muriel took a seat. To her immediate left was a bookcase, so I positioned myself between the two adjacent seats. Once again Beth Stein performed the magical needle work and got Muriel hooked up to an IV. There was no blood draw today, just the infusion of the 90 mg of Aredia over a 90-minute period. I had brought in the Phase 10 cards and we proceeded to while away the time playing the game. I did all the necessary shuffling and dealing as Muriel had one hand pretty well tied up with the IV. The distraction of the card game made the time go by quickly and we were soon on our way home. There has been no indication of how long these treatments will go on, but I guess if there are holes in the bones they will need to be filled. I certainly wouldn't want Muriel to fall and experience broken limbs in addition to everything else. After I got Muriel home I went and hit a bucket of golf balls in preparation for the start of the golfing season.

Friday, May 4, 2001

This is a quite significant day in the history of northern Ohio, and particularly at Kent State University. It marks the 31st anniversary of the deaths of four students on their campus during a protest of the Vietnam War. It also was a traumatic day in our lives as I was on campus that day and Muriel was at work in her job as 7th grade teacher in the Hudson Public Schools. We didn't have cell phones back then and were thus at the mercy of the land line system. Muriel tried to get in touch with me to confirm I was all right, but with so many people calling in and calling out all she ever got was a busy signal. She had no idea whether I was still on campus or whether I had come home. All she knew for sure was I had left home that morning to teach my class and then to attend my doctoral class in human resources with professor Robert D. Smith. It wasn't until she came home from teaching and found me at home that she breathed a sigh of relief. However, today I wasn't going to a class and Muriel wasn't teaching. We were just going to an appointment with Dr. Doncals in the radiation therapy department. It was the two-week follow-up from the last visit. Dr. Doncals greeted us and directed Muriel to be seated on the examination table. She immediately began asking questions. "Are you having any pain in the pelvic area?"

"Right now I am pain-free. I haven't taken any pills for pain in weeks. My only complaint is the occurrence of diarrhea."

"Do you think it could be affected by what you are eating?"

"I don't really know. My appetite has been good and I have even gained some weight."

"I have literature on a low residue diet. Please read it over and keep track of the foods that you think might be triggering the diarrhea."

"All right. All I know is that right now, taking two Lomotil and one Kadian just shuts it right down."

"Well, continue to do that until we can figure this out."

When Dr. Doncals completed her examination, I made an appointment for Muriel for June and we left for home.

Saturday, May 5, 2001

We are getting ready to go away again for a week, and today we are making some of the necessary preparations for that trip. One of the things I did was mow the lawn because it is not going to be done for a week. We partially packed the car and then went to Outback Steakhouse for dinner. I had a Foster's and Muriel settled for a glass of Merlot. My main dish was the barbecued ribs with fries while Muriel had the petite steak with a baked potato. Muriel continues to be very upbeat about her adventure, so I was surprised tonight when she shared her initial reservations about the radiation treatments.

"When I first started the radiation treatments and nothing happened after the first three, I was just a little skeptical that the pain was not going to go away. But it was about that time that I noticed when I lifted my leg I had no pain."

"You never said anything to me about that."

"I didn't want you to worry unnecessarily because there was *some* improvement. It just wasn't as fast as I wanted it to be."

"I know you are the one who is carrying the burden, but I would hope you would share your thoughts with me so I can help find answers to your concerns."

"Well I have a concern right now and that's this diarrhea. I know I can treat it effectively with the meds but it's annoying that it keeps recurring."

"Maybe it's time to see Dr. Cline. I think that Dr. Doncals and Dr. Abood would agree that you do that. The next time you see Dr. Koenig, ask him what he thinks."

After dinner we went to E. J. Thomas Hall where we were entertained by the Akron Symphony Orchestra. Ya-Hui Wang once again was the conductor and selected Leonard Bernstein's "Three Dance Episodes" from *On the Town* to begin the program. It was a lively way to begin the evening. Ravel was the composer for the next two pieces, Piano Concerto for the Left Hand in D Major and Piano Concerto in G Major, with Pascal Rogé as the solo pianist. I recognized the former piece from an episode of M*A*S*H. The storyline was the injury to the right hand of a budding concert pianist. Of course, he was despondent and Major Winchester tried to cheer him up by providing him with Ravel's piece for the left hand. Major Winchester was judged as being condescending by the soldier, but he left the music anyway. The scene dissolves to the piano in the recreation tent with the pianist playing the piece for the left hand and the viewers were happy. We, too, were happy with the performances of Mr. Rogé. The program closed with *The Firebird* Suite by Stravinsky. Fifteen minutes after the concert ended we were home in Munroe Falls, far better than that long trip from Cleveland.

Sunday, May 13, 2001

On May 6th we left Munroe Falls at 4:00 in the morning and drove to Edisto Beach in South Carolina. We had reserved a time-share week and we were assigned to the facility that was right on the ocean. Unlike Myrtle Beach, Edisto Beach is non-commercial. As a result one can walk the beaches and not see anyone for long stretches. We were located right at the entrance to an inlet and could watch the comings and goings of the small boats that were moored in the marina. Each day we took our beach chairs and staked out an area as our home base where we just basked in the sun, read books, and watched the dolphins that cavorted in the ocean. Periodically, hand in hand, we would take long walks along the beach. There was no great need for conversation as we watched the gulls circle and land only to take flight again minutes later. There is a certain smell that is present at the ocean, and I am beginning to like it nearly as much as Muriel. We had a sensitivity toward each other that precluded breaking the stillness of the situation.

I played golf a couple of times, and we attended an old-fashioned "low country boil" for the first time in our lives. The shrimp, corn, sausage, and red potatoes were all boiled together in a huge pot. When it was deemed to be done the pot was drained and all of the goodies were dumped onto a huge table from which we served ourselves. The shrimp were cooked with the shells on so there was a little work involved in the meal, but it was well worth it as everything tasted so delicious. Many of us had seconds as we wanted to make sure that nothing edible was left on the table. It was a great week and this evening we returned to Munroe Falls reinvigorated. Muriel has a determination that she can handle whatever comes her way as we return to our regular routine.

Monday, May 21, 2001

This morning we returned to Dr. Koenig's office for another Aredia treatment and to have Muriel see the doctor. We didn't have to wait long as we were among the first ones into the office. Muriel was weighed (131 pounds) and had her blood pressure taken (122/78). Dr. Koenig seemed pleased with Muriel's progress, although he has a continuing concern for her intermittent diarrhea. He also indicated that he wanted her to have both a bone scan and a CT scan later in the summer. She was cleared for her Aredia treatment so we moved from the examination room to the chemotherapy room. This time Muriel was seated in the chair just before the seat in the alcove. After Beth got the IV positioned I sat on a stool right next to her chair. I asked, "Why didn't you ask Dr. Koenig about seeing Dr. Cline?"

"When he said he wanted me to have a bone scan and a CT scan he mentioned that the results might provide some clues as to why I was having diarrhea."

"But he wants those scans later in summer. What about now?"

"I can treat it with the meds for now until we see him again."

"If you think that's best then that's what we'll do." We played a game of Phase 10 and then read while the 90 minutes elapsed.

Friday, June 1, 2001

We begin the month with a trip to the radiation therapy department and an appointment with Dr. Doncals. It represents another follow-up session to the radiation therapy that she completed in February.

I don't recall that there were as many follow-ups when Muriel had the first radiation therapy in March of 1999. I suspect the increased frequency has to do with the study that Muriel agreed to be a part of, as she continues to complete questionnaires on each visit. Once again Dr. Doncals was her usual ebullient self and treated us like long lost friends. She had a myriad of questions for Muriel and performed her usual examination. As for the diarrhea, Dr. Doncals recommended that Muriel try a daily dose of Imodium to see if this will ease the attacks.

Monday, June 11, 2001

Muriel was not awake when I left for Bible class and then went on to play golf with my usual Monday morning foursome. However, I had left the traveling birthday card, as well as an additional note expressing my love for her, on the kitchen table that would greet her when she came down for her morning coffee. Today Muriel catches up with me and turns 66. She was up when I returned from golf and I wished her a happy birthday in person and gave her my present. I had lunch and then worked for a while in the backyard. By then it was time to shower and get ready for our date. We went to The Olive Garden for dinner. We had no difficulty getting a seat in the non-smoking section and began our dinner with a glass of wine. While we ate salad and breadsticks the conversation drifted to the status of Muriel's adventure.

"I have accepted the fact that I am no longer cancer-free," she said.

"And what does that mean?" I asked.

"It means it's no longer a case of living a full life but garnering as many years together as we can."

"Bah humbug! We don't know what God has in store for us. He gave you peace at the outset and He has been known to perform miracles. He probably has one ready for you. That's what I keep praying for."

"Thank you sweetheart. But, as I told you before, I hope I make it to our 50th wedding anniversary. That would be a great, and then God can take me home."

"I won't be ready for you to go home then. I think you should hang around 'til our 60th."

"Okay, I'll do that," she said with a big grin on her face.

It was the first time I sensed a chink in her armor but the smile at the end told me she remains positive, trusting that God will see her through this. Our main course arrived and, as we both began to eat, Muriel said, "I know I have said this before, but I want you to promise me that if I have further metastases you will do whatever it takes to have me remain pain-free."

"I can make that promise, but I think you have to let me be the judge regarding my intervention if and when you have additional metastases and become incapacitated."

"I'm also concerned that you are doing far too much for me and not doing the things you enjoy, like playing bridge and golfing."

"Hey, that's why I retired, so I could take care of you."

"C'mon, be serious."

"I am serious. Way back on a cold night in January I promised before God and all those assembled that I would care for you in sickness and in health, and right now sickness is center stage. Be assured my dear, I will golf, I will play bridge, and I will ski. But you have to let me be the judge of when I do that."

"I know sweetheart. It's just that when you do those things you always come back invigorated and I want you to have those opportunities."

"I will assure you that there will be a time when I will have Lois in to care for you, or maybe even home health care so I can go out knowing you are in good hands. I have maintained a long-term health care policy for you so I'll get it out and see what we are eligible for." We finished our dinner, shared a tiramisu for dessert, and then went home and watched *The Mask of Zorro*.

Monday, June 18, 2001

Since the time we saw Dr. Doncals at the beginning of the month, our lives are pretty much back to the status quo. Muriel is doing the cooking, taking care of the washing and ironing, preparing shopping lists, and preparing for the upcoming Chorale season. I am playing golf on Mondays and Wednesdays, continuing to work in the backyard, and running whatever errands need to be run. In addition to the regular support group meetings that Muriel attends, she and three of the other regulars—Robin, Linda, and Sue—meet for lunch once during the month. These three together with Muriel have become very close. Muriel is the oldest of the group, and I judge the others look up to her with awe in the way she has handled all of the ramifications of her disease. I don't think that Muriel has ever been envious of the other three, but it could be easy to be that way considering that none of the others have had a metastasis of the breast cancer.

Today our daughter and her children, Kaitlyn and Kenton, arrived from Texas to spend the week with us. Although Kay and her children spend time with us at our time-share week in North Myrtle Beach, it is a rare occasion for either of our children to return home to Ohio to visit. When the grandkids were small it was much easier for Grandpa and Oma to travel to Texas. From the time each grandchild became five, they were allowed to come and spend a week with us during the summertime. We would go to Cedar Point and Sea World and spoil them rotten. One year we had all three of them (Emma Catherine was not yet born) at the same time. We called it Camp Klafehn, and Muriel made T-shirts for each of them with their names across the back. We had a good time together, although there were some conflicts between the cousins. It was the only time we had all three simultaneously.

One of the main reasons they had come to Ohio this time was to visit Cedar Point. Kay had worked at the amusement park for two summers while she was in college and barely had any time off to go on the rides. Cedar Point is famed for the number and variety of roller coasters they have. Kay had issued a challenge to each of her kids to ride all of the coasters with mom, so a trip to Cedar Point was planned later in the week.

Tuesday, June 19, 2001

While our daughter and grandchildren slept in, Muriel and I went to Dr. Koenig's office for an examination and another Aredia treatment. We parked on the second floor of the parking deck enabling us to walk right to Dr. Koenig's office without having to take an elevator up or down. We blended in with the crowd and while Muriel completed some paperwork, I perused a section of the *Akron Beacon Journal*. We were soon ushered into the inner sanctum where Muriel was weighed (128½ pounds) and she was then brought to the examination room to have her blood pressure taken (118/68). As usual, Muriel supplied the nurse with an up-to-date list of her medications. Next came the paper blouse and the wait for Dr. Koenig. He arrived and asked the usual questions followed by an examination. Muriel indicated she was having difficulty sleeping and asked Dr. Koenig if he would be willing to give her a prescription for Valium. I can't know his mind, but he always seemed to look at having his patient be most comfortable whatever the circumstances, so he provided her with a prescription for 5 mg of Valium. Dr. Koenig reiterated that he wanted Muriel to repeat the CT and bone scans at the end of the month or in August.

We left the examination room and moved to the chemotherapy room where Muriel was fortunate enough to get the chair in the alcove.

Beth was busy with another patient so Ruth Clark put in the IV. This time it was in the wrist. Oftentimes this location for the needle had been difficult because of "vein rolls" but Ruth had no difficulty. I had brought the Phase 10 cards and we played a game. Muriel trounced me and I was eager to play again, but she decided that we would end on a positive note for her, and that was okay with me. After 90 minutes the IV was removed and we headed back to the car.

By the time we got home Kay and her family were up and we all had lunch together. After lunch, Kay, Kenton, Kaitlyn, and I all went out to Fox Den Golf Course to play golf. Kay and Kenton had brought their clubs with them and Kaitlyn used Muriel's clubs. Kaitlyn had never played before and she did more riding of the golf cart than she did hitting the ball. It was a nice outing for the four of us, and when we returned Muriel had prepared a picnic dinner for us all. We all showered, loaded the car, and headed for Goodyear Heights Metro Park where the Akron Symphony Orchestra was giving a free summer open-air concert. We had our dinner on the lawn and then moved our chairs into position for the concert. Many of the regulars had the summer off and the orchestra was supplemented with musicians from the music departments of both Kent State University and the University of Akron. We had brought insect repellent so we were well-prepared for the mosquito brigade when it arrived. We all had a good time.

Thursday, June 21, 2001

This morning we piled into Kay's Lincoln Navigator and headed to Cedar Point in Sandusky, Ohio. I had the privilege of driving that big old monstrosity. One is seated so high off the ground that it is like driving a semi. It took a little getting used to for me, but we survived the trip. We bought two-day tickets as I had made reservations to stay at the Comfort Inn in Sandusky for the night. The roller coaster challenge began immediately, as just inside the park gates is the Raptor. It is an inverted coaster in which you are seated in a suspended chair and looped and rolled and whipped around corners, not to mention the initial drop. With the exception of Muriel, who found a comfortable bench to sit on, the rest of us snaked our way through the Disney-like maze waiting area until we reached the loading platform after about a 45-minute wait. Later on in the day as the park became more crowded, the waiting times increased significantly. We all rode the Sky Ride in suspended gondolas from which one gets an overall view of the park. The ride ends near the Cedar Point & Lake Erie Railroad train station.

We took a ride on one of the trains over to Frontiertown and rode several more roller coasters. One was the Cedar Creek Mine Ride, a very smooth ride that ends with a double helix pulling a lot of g's as you enter the station and come to a braking stop. Next was White Water Landing, a log flume water ride that gave us an opportunity to cool off as the final plunge down a water chute results in a huge splash that sends water cascading back over the passengers. Kenton just loved the Giant Swing, which consists of chairs on long chains anchored at the top to a center stack that begins to slowly turn, swinging the chairs further and further out due to the centrifugal action. Fortunately there was not a long line as he went back several times. Another wet ride we enjoyed was Thunder Canyon, where a huge inner tube with seats moves through a waterway passing many locations where there are waterfalls. Since the tube twirls as it moves through the waterway there were many opportunities to get further drenched.

We rode on many rides that Muriel could also be a part of such as Cedar Downs Racing Derby, a type of carousel, and three car-track rides named Cadillac Cars, Turnpike Cars, and Antique Cars. We ate funnel cake, popcorn, and soft ice cream. I participated in additional roller coaster rides including Gemini, Iron Dragon, Corkscrew, and the old classic wooden roller coaster named Blue Streak, the oldest operating coaster in the park. Kaitlyn and Muriel rode Scrambler together several times. We wrapped up the day around four o'clock and checked into the motel. There was a nice big pool so we switched to our bathing suits and extended our fun time. We went to dinner at Denny's where everyone was happy that they served breakfast around the clock. There was no problem falling asleep this night.

Friday, June 22, 2001

We were up early and had breakfast at the motel. We then returned to the park for another day of fun. One of the coasters we rode today was called Disaster Transport. You go through three different buildings as you work your way through the maze. Again, we got to this ride at a good time and had a minimal wait. It is totally indoors and in total darkness except for strobe effects. It is a little scary. Kenton and I rode the Mean Streak and WildCat coasters. Kay and Kaitlyn also rode them, as well as the Magnum XL-200 and Millennium Force coasters. We all rode the Paddlewheel Excursions boat and the Midway Carousel. The last coaster the four of us rode is called the Mantis. It is unusual in that we stood in individual cages, but at least we didn't go upside down.

We played "crash" in the Dodgem cars. The Witches' Wheel was nearly a disaster for my stomach. Each rider is in an individual capsule-like car. The ride begins on the horizontal and slowly tilts upward as it goes around and around and around. I was extremely happy to get off of that ride. You would have thought I'd learned my lesson, but we then chose three more spinning rides, Matterhorn, Calypso, and a ride named Chaos. That ride is interesting as two people ride in a capsule-like carriage that flips completely over in either a forward or backward roll as the ride rotates and tilts the individual capsules. The backward roll was very disorienting but my stomach again managed to contain itself. And as if that wasn't enough, we ate more junk food!

We stayed around for the laser show and fireworks and then headed home. Kay was kind enough to drive us home as we laughed and giggled all the way, recalling each of the rides and the feelings we had in riding them. Even though Muriel didn't ride as many rides as the rest of us, while we were off doing our thing she people watched, one of her favorite pastimes. Tomorrow, we will bid goodbye to them all as they head back to Texas, but when we arrived at the motel Kay decided she would pack the car in the morning for their return trip. Like the night before, there was no difficulty falling asleep.

Tuesday, July 3, 2001

Should one consider a visit to the doctor a pre-holiday trip? Whether you do or not that was our agenda for the day, another follow-up session with Dr. Doncals, Muriel's radiation oncologist. It had been two weeks since her visit to Dr. Koenig and the diarrhea had not abated, so Muriel arrived with the goal of getting some definitive answers. She greeted us and asked Muriel, "How are you doing?"

"Not so good. I have no bone pain but the occurrences of diarrhea have increased, as has the accompanying abdominal pain. I can't go out of the house for fear I will have an accident. This just can't go on."

"Last time we met you were going to keep track of things you were eating that might have triggered the diarrhea. Did you discover anything?"

"I don't think food has anything to do with it. I realize that Lomotil and Kadian shut it down but I would like a solution to the problem, not a stopgap measure."

"I understand your concern and I'm sorry for all of your discomfort. I would like to talk with Dr. Koenig and maybe we can agree on a course of action."

After Dr. Doncals stepped out of the room I said, "Wow, you are your feisty self this morning."

"Well, I've had enough. The two of them don't have to live with this, but I do and I'm sick and tired of it."

Dr. Doncals returned and began talking as she came through the door. "The first thing we want you to do is to stop taking the Arimidex. You are also taking a variety of vitamins and supplements and we want you to stop taking those as well. There is no guarantee that this will stop the diarrhea, but it will allow us to rule out some things we think may be triggering it. We also want you to provide a stool sample which we will send out to be analyzed."

After Dr. Doncals completed her physical examination of Muriel we left for home. As we walked to the car I asked Muriel, "Do you think their plan to tackle this is going to help?"

"I'm not sure, but at least there seems to be an effort to solve it."

Wednesday, July 4, 2001

We walked over to Route 59 in Stow and watched the annual Fourth of July parade. There were several floats and bands, the Tadmor Temple motorcyclists, convertibles with celebrities and politicians, fire department marchers, and the ubiquitous fire and rescue trucks with their sirens doing a slow whine. I never could figure out why it was really necessary to blow the sirens, as it raised havoc with the ears of the elderly—and others as well—and generally frightened many of the small children. Even if they did throw candy to the spectators it was inappropriate. Why not just ring the bell? We quietly spent the rest of the day and enjoyed a picnic meal indoors.

Saturday, July 7, 2001

Soon after Muriel began taking Valium for her insomnia, she no longer had issues with her sleep. Last night was no exception so she awoke early and well-rested. It was the first Saturday of the month and thus the day of her support group meeting, but the day was to begin with a grocery shopping trip. Because of Kay's visit last month, we had meals left over and had delayed our usual early-in-the-month shopping excursion. It was always easier to go during the week when stores would not be as crowded, but the list had not been ready until late Thursday and yesterday I was at the Bridgestone Invitational. Before going to Tops for groceries we stopped off at BJ's, a bulk discount store, to pick-up some economy-sized cans of mixed nuts and any other items that might have piqued our interest. We rarely have a list when we go to BJ's, and let our impulses take over. However, we did maintain a reasonable measure of self-control. Muriel was out for the afternoon at her support group, and I spent the time watching the usual sporting fare on TV. In the evening we went to the Blossom Music Center where we were treated to several lush musical pieces by the Cleveland Orchestra performing under the baton of Steven Smith, the assistant conductor of the orchestra.

Tuesday, July 17, 2001

We had a morning appointment in Dr. Koenig's office for a follow-up visit and to have Muriel's Aredia treatment. I was surprised that the waiting room was not jammed and we were called in almost immediately. Muriel was weighed (128½ pounds) and then had her blood pressure taken (120/70). Dr. Koenig asked Muriel about the diarrhea and she indicated it was still occurring every three to five days, and not taking supplements or vitamins had no effect. She also told him she had been off all medications for a while and that there were no positive cultures found in the stool sample. Dr. Koenig completed a physical examination of Muriel, then suggested she go back on the Arimidex and the other medications and supplements she had stopped. He also reiterated that he wanted Muriel to have a new bone scan and a CT scan toward the end of the month or early next month. I told him I would speak with his scheduling person and take care of it.

Next came the Aredia treatment. No corner chair today and again Ruth Clark was able to find a vein in Muriel's wrist to set up the IV. Initially she drew a vial of blood, and then began the Aredia infusion. When Muriel was squared away, I went to speak with the scheduling clerk and set up the two scans that Dr. Koenig wanted Muriel to have. The clerk made the necessary calls and we ended up with a CT scan of the chest, abdomen, and pelvis, with contrast at 9:30 on July 26th. The whole body bone scan was also scheduled for 9:30 but would not take place until August 9th. Having accomplished that, I returned to the chemotherapy room and took up my usual place on the stool by Muriel's chair. I had brought the Phase 10 cards but Muriel was content to just read as the remainder of the 90 minutes passed by. We had a light lunch after we got home and then I went and hit a bucket of balls while Muriel relaxed in the family room.

Monday, July 23, 2001

This morning I went to my breakfast Bible class and then on to my usual round of golf. After lunch we took a trip into Akron City

Hospital to pre-register Muriel for her CT scan. We decided that it was easier to pre-register and cope with the bureaucracy during an uncritical time rather than wait until the morning of the test. Actually, all went smoothly, and now we would be able to go straight to the department where the CT scan was to be administered.

Thursday, July 26, 2001

I was up early and exercised, and then we were off for Muriel's CT scan. We parked in the deck and walked across the street and directly to the X-ray department. Muriel checked in and they were aware that she was pre-registered. We had just settled into our chairs when the CT technician called us to the room where the scan was to take place. I stayed with Muriel while they put in an IV, and then I was shooed off to the CT scan waiting area. About an hour later the nurse came to get me. The CT scan was complete and we were set to go. We walked back to the parking deck and began to make our way home.

"Today was a B+," Muriel said.

"That's good." The grade was Muriel's mark for the level of pain she had to endure while the nurse or technician was trying to find a vein. She still thinks that Beth Stein, one of Dr. Koenig's nurses, is the best.

Thursday, August 2, 2001

Four months have passed since our last visit to Dr. Abood in Kent. We were called into an examination room soon after we arrived and Dottie checked Muriel's weight (138 pounds), blood pressure (115/70), temperature (97.9°) and pulse (80). Dottie also asked about her pain level and Muriel indicated a five on a scale of one to ten. However, she also qualified that, confining it to the times she has had the diarrhea and cramping. This was the second time that Muriel had seen Dr. Abood since the metastasis to the bone and the additional radiation. He was aware that she had been hospitalized shortly after the completion of the radiation. He was very concerned about her continuing problem with the diarrhea and cramping. He noted that it was four months that this has been going on. They talked about the Lomotil and the Kadian, the stool samples, the absence of medications and supplements, and then reintroducing them one by one. He suggested that she may want to consult a GI specialist. However, she didn't want to do that until she got the results from the newest bone and CT scans. He asked if she was using her puffers on a regular basis, and I verified that she was not only doing it on a regular basis, but was recording the number of puffs she was doing each time. He noted that she had lost nine pounds since the last time she was there. Muriel figured most of it had to do with the diarrhea, but she also admitted that her appetite was somewhat off. He suggested she call if the symptoms became more severe and that she should return in two months. He also wanted her to have a blood test, which she did at the outpatient lab of Robinson Memorial Hospital.

Friday, August 3, 2001

I was away most of the day playing in a golf outing to benefit Lutheran Children's Aid & Family Services. While I was out Muriel called Dr. Doncals to see if she had any further suggestions regarding her intermittent bouts of diarrhea. The doctor cited a study regarding the use of vitamin E, so Muriel is now embarking on this regimen. All of the diarrhea problems began upon completion of radiation therapy back in April, so we are now entering the fifth month and I judge it is beginning to weigh heavily on Muriel's resolve.

Thursday, August 9, 2001

It was back to the hospital today for Muriel's bone scan. This is the one where you have an initial test and go home, and then later in the day you return for another test. Between tests there is a need to drink lots of water to flush the system. Adding extra liquid to Muriel's fragile system was probably not the best thing going, but she was a good trooper and tried to meet the challenge.

Friday, August 17, 2001

On the morning of August 10th, we were off to North Myrtle Beach and a week at the ocean. As we have taken this trip for so many years and have driven there so many times, my car can almost get us there automatically. We always start very early in the morning so that we arrive late afternoon, have a quick dinner, and spend time walking on the beach in the evening. Kay and her family joined us again. We were blessed with a week of sunshine, and Kay, Kenton, and I played golf three times, while Muriel and Kaitlyn sat on the beach. We worked on the usual jigsaw puzzle, played Phase 10 and UNO, and went out to eat toward the end of our stay. Kay and Muriel each provided three meals, and with Walmart right up the road from us, we got all of the necessary staples that we needed for the week. Even though she was plagued with the diarrhea bug, Muriel is always bolstered by a trip to the ocean. Each evening at dusk we would walk hand in hand on the beach, sometimes on the sand and other times in the wash of the waves, returning to the condo well after the sun had set. I can almost sense a surge in energy as Muriel is exposed to that environment. She reiterated that when she dies she wishes to be cremated and have her ashes strewn at the ocean. Not knowing when that will happen, we squeezed our hands a little tighter in the foreshadowing of that moment. Despite the long day spent journeying home, we arrived in Munoe Falls well-rested Friday evening.

Saturday, August 18, 2001

Every time we go away there is some catching up to do when we get back. Today was that kind of a day. My neighbor, Scott, was kind enough to mow our front lawn while we were away, and I judged the back lawn could wait a few more days. I got the golf cards from the previous week's play and spent some time getting all of the statistics in order for the coming week. I picked up the mail and sorted through everything. It is always amazing to me that when we return from a week or more away from home that we have accumulated a hamper full of mail. So the sorting, slitting, and dividing of the mail—Muriel's pile and my pile—took nearly a half hour.

Then there was the need to sort through and discard all of the superfluous mail, which generally filled the recycle bin. Muriel's pile consisted mainly of catalogs. She is a great telephone shopper and, of course, the catalog is the vehicle that gets the customer in the door. Some of her favorites are Eddie Bauer, J. Jill, Talbots, L.L.Bean, and many video catalogs. As catalog houses are wont to do, they sell their subscriber list to other catalog houses and a new wave of catalogs comes to our doorstep. In anticipation of Muriel's death, I had cataloged her catalogs, planning for a systematic cancellation of them all when the time came. Remarkably, I compiled a list of 108 companies that have been sending her catalogs. My plan is to maintain a record of each call I will make and the person to whom I speak. If another catalog is to come, I will call back to confirm cancellation (some of Muriel's organizational skills rubbed off on me).

In the evening we went to the Blossom Music Center for the Cleveland Orchestra concert. We had seats in the pavilion, and the performance included "The Walk to the Paradise Garden" from the Frederick Delius opera *A Village Romeo and Juliet*, "Songs of a Wayfarer" by Mahler, and Mozart's Mass in C Minor. All were under the direction of Sir Andrew Davis. It was a hot and sticky night, but the music minimized any discomfort as it wafted through the pavilion and on out to those patrons on the lawn beyond.

Tuesday, August 28, 2001

Muriel had an appointment with Dr. Koenig this morning. It was a six-week follow-up to her last appointment and we were to find out the results of the CT scan and the full body scan. She was also scheduled to have an Aredia treatment. There was nearly a full house in the waiting room but we were quickly ushered in where Muriel was weighed (124½ pounds) and then taken to an examination room where the nurse took her blood pressure (126/70). Dr. Koenig arrived in an upbeat mood as he was happy to report that the scans indicated no new tumors. He had compared the new scans to the scans taken earlier in the year. Muriel reiterated for the umpteenth time that she was still suffering from the diarrhea. Dr. Koenig suggested that she try psyllium husk powder. All sorts of precautions were given, as the powder is intended to absorb liquid and assist in forming a solid stool. At this point Muriel was happy to try anything that might provide relief.

Dr. Koenig performed a physical examination and then we crossed to the chemotherapy room for the 90-minute session of Aredia infusion. Beth Stein had no problem finding a vein in Muriel's hand and all went well with the needle stick and IV. We played Phase 10 again today and finished the game just prior to the completion of the treatment. On the way home we stopped at New Earth to pick up the psyllium husk powder. Sue Wells was not working, so we were in and out and quickly back to 87 Oakhurst Drive.

Sunday, September 23, 2001

The information that Muriel had gotten from Dr. Koenig at the end of August, i.e., no new lesions, carried us into the month of September and our lives returned to normal, or as normal as can be when one of those persons has their life hanging in the balance. But Muriel is not about to throw in the towel, as she soldiers on. I shouldn't use that metaphor as it implies a battle and she would be appalled that I would even allude to her battling cancer.

We began to hike the Metro Park trails as we worked for another medallion on our hiking staffs. We also spent another week at Edisto Beach in South Carolina. It was a peaceful and carefree time, and both of us read several books during the week. We once again attended the low country boil. Having been to our first in May, going to another was on our "must-do" list and this time around was equally enjoyable. Once you have gone to one of those outings, you don't want to miss the next one.

Tuesday, September 25, 2001

This was a tripleheader day. We started with an initial visit to Dr. Koenig at 9:45, followed by an appointment with Dr. Doncals at 10:30, and then back for an Aredia treatment at 1:00. We parked in the parking deck and walked into the physician's office building, and then took the elevator up to the second floor. The waiting room was once again close to capacity. I often forget that Summit Oncology is a practice that has three oncologists and that there are bound to be several patients coming and going. Muriel was weighed (130½ pounds) and had her blood pressure taken (150/80). Dr. Koenig asked whether the psyllium husk powder had any effect on the diarrhea and the answer, unfortunately, had to be no. He indicated that he was going to give her a prescription for Questran. I don't think Muriel has reached the desperation stage and is willing to try anything that might relieve her of the every-third-day diarrhea. He did a physical examination and we left with an appointment for next month.

We left Dr. Koenig's office with the new prescription for Questran, crossed the bridge on the second floor, and took the elevator to the first floor where our next stop was the radiation therapy department for a date with Dr. Doncals. The question of the diarrhea was the first thing she asked about, and Muriel indicated that the increase in vitamin E as well as vitamin C, together with the psyllium husk powder Dr. Koenig suggested, had no effect, and that Dr. Koenig had now given her a prescription for Questran. Muriel was concerned that nothing had worked and stated that she was ready to go back to see Dr. Cline, her gastroenterologist. Dr. Doncals readily agreed. The physical examination was similar to the one she had just been given by Dr. Koenig except for the addition of the strength measurement.

It was after 11:00 when we left the examination area of the radiation therapy department and I said, "Let's go to the hospital cafeteria and have lunch."

"I don't want to go to the cafeteria."

"Well, that leaves us McDonald's or the Country Kitchen. Do you want to order from the menu or do fast food?"

"I want to go to the Country Kitchen."

We decided to walk over as it was a pleasant day. We were seated in a booth and I ordered a bacon, lettuce, and tomato sandwich on whole wheat. Muriel had a sliced turkey sandwich with lettuce and tomato on rye. We each had a Diet Pepsi and shared an order of fries. We had a nice leisurely lunch and mulled over Muriel's bowel problems, a luncheon conversation that only we could find appropriate. We are amazed that three doctors have been trying to solve her problem to no avail, a problem that has gone on for nearly a half year. Fortunately, she has the Kadian that at least shuts everything down for a few days. Maybe Dr. Cline can make a determination.

At 12:30 we headed back to Dr. Koenig's office for Muriel's Aredia treatment. When we arrived we were the only ones in the chemotherapy room, so Muriel chose the seat in the alcove and Beth Stein set up the IV in her left arm. We both read while we waited for the infusion to be complete. Back in 1998 when all of this was new to us, we were eager to talk with others and to share experiences. However, as time has passed—incidentally, today marks the third anniversary of the initial diagnosis—we are less likely to engage others in conversation. We are not reluctant to talk, but we do not seek out others during these times as we did in the past. We make the judgment that others do not want to hear about metastasis, particularly if they are in their first round of chemotherapy which they are hoping will kill all of the cancer cells so that each individual can get back to a regular life. Perhaps some of it also has to do with the fact that each time Muriel has had an Aredia treatment, nearly all of the people in the room are different from the last time we were there. So we read or play Phase 10 and we become ships that pass in the night. When the Aredia infusion was completed we made our way home. Upon our arrival, I made a call to Dr. Cline's office to set up an appointment for November 7th. It had been a long day, but after dinner we went off to Chorale practice where Muriel was her usual effervescent self as she rehearsed the Chorale through several pieces.

Tuesday, October 2, 2001

Muriel and I traveled to Kent this morning for a regular check-up with her internist, Dr. Abood. Dottie took all of the vital statistics: weight (128 pounds), blood pressure (126/68), temperature (99°), and pulse (80). The first thing he asked about was the diarrhea and Muriel had to inform him that there had been no change, and further, that she had made an appointment with Dr. Cline for November. Dr. Abood also agreed that seeing a gastroenterologist was a good idea. She also let him know that the latest bone and CT scans were clear of any new tumors. He asked about her shoulder which she had complained about the last time she had visited, and Muriel indicated that the pain had gone away on its own. He did a physical examination and provided her with renewal prescriptions for some of the medications she is taking on a regular basis. He also gave her an order to have blood drawn at the laboratory right in the building. He suggested we should return in three months.

We made an appointment for January 3rd of next year, and departed for the hematology laboratory on the first floor where Muriel had blood drawn. Apparently the lady who does this blood work is nearly as good as Beth Stein in Dr. Koenig's office. Whenever she has blood drawn in the Kent facility, I have not been allowed to accompany her. It is one of the very few places where I have not been able to sit and hold her hand while she gets stuck, or listen to the comments of the doctors or nurses. We wished that hadn't been the case since we had decided right from the start of Muriel's adventure that two sets of ears were better than one, and oftentimes we would review what we each had heard on any given occasion.

Monday, October 29, 2001

The rest of the month was typical for us. We shopped for groceries for the month at Tops Foods. We hiked more of the Metro Park trails and were able to again secure our medallions. We turned in our list before we had completed all 13 this year as Muriel judged that the trails rated three were too strenuous for her. We called Dr. Koenig's office in the middle of the month and indicated that Muriel had been taking one packet of Questran daily and it was doing no good. He suggested that she increase it to two. We went to the Akron Civic Theatre for Ohio Ballet, and to E. J. Thomas Hall where we heard the second concert of the year by the Akron Symphony Orchestra. We were soothed by Ottorino Respighi's *Pines of Rome*, Debussy's *La Mer*, and a wonderful piece by Joaquín Rodrigo entitled *Concierto de Aranjuez* with Christopher Parkening on solo guitar.

I checked the Internet to see if there was anything with regard to the side effects of pelvic radiation. I found nothing, though perhaps I didn't look in the right places. We called our granddaughter Emma Catherine and sang "Happy Birthday" to her—it was her third—and carried on a pleasant but one-sided conversation with her as she jabbered away.

Tuesday, October 30, 2001

Today we headed back to Dr. Koenig's office for a follow-up visit. We were able to park on the second floor of the parking deck and thus, able to walk directly to Dr. Koenig's office. We did not wait long before we were ushered into the preexamination area where Muriel was weighed (123½ pounds), and then to the examination room where she had her blood pressure taken (118/66). When Dr. Koenig came in, the topic of conversation quickly turned to the state of the diarrhea. Muriel reported that Questran had no effect and she had made an appointment to see Dr. Cline. There wasn't too much to discuss after that, so he examined her and prepared to send her off for an Aredia treatment. He suggested that we follow-up in one month, but Muriel informed him that we would be in Tennessee for a week, and then on out to Colorado for approximately three weeks. She wanted to know if not having an Aredia treatment in a month would cause her any additional problems. He assured her it would not and that he would see us in five to six weeks, whatever is convenient for us.

Wednesday, October 31, 2001

It is the end of the month and my birthday. I now moved past Muriel once again to 67. Muriel passed on the joint card and a gift of Stetson Cologne, one of my favorites. We whiled away the afternoon by going to the movies. Yes, we still go out to see movies even though we have over 600 videos in the house.

Saturday, November 3, 2001

This morning I did the Heart Walk wearing my red hat as one of the honorees. I have been walking in the Heart Walk every year since I had open heart surgery, so today marks the 17th time I have participated.

< 10 >
SOLVING THE DIARRHEA DILEMMA

Wednesday, November 7, 2001

Today, after seven months of episodic diarrhea, Muriel saw Dr. Cline at Digestive Health Services. Muriel explained what has transpired in her life since she had last seen him. Of course, the emphasis was on the diarrhea, originally diagnosed as radiation enteritis. Dr. Cline did a complete examination of Muriel and concluded he would have a better idea of her problem and how to deal with it if she had another colonoscopy. She told him we would be out of town until the 9th of December, so he scheduled her colonoscopy for December 19th. Before we left, Dr. Cline suggested she continue to use the Lomotil and Kadian to shut down the diarrhea.

Thursday, November 8, 2001

We spent the day preparing for an extended vacation and taking care of all of the loose ends that are inevitable when you are preparing to travel. I even had some time left over to rake leaves for a couple of hours. I don't know how many books Muriel packed, but I had five books and three puzzles. It was the first time that I had packed both my golf clubs and my skis on the same trip. When you are away for four weeks you are not in a position to take along prepared meals, so we packed spices according to the recipes that Muriel had selected for our stay and anticipated buying the main ingredients at the different locations where we would be staying. One of the things we will take with us is a frozen turkey, anticipating that we can roast it after it has thawed and then proceed to have turkey sandwiches, turkey stir-fry, and other meals where turkey would be the base.

Monday, December 10, 2001

Early on Friday, November 9th, we left for Fairfield Glade. Driving to Fairfield Glade in Tennessee is not a problem, and with the change into Central Daylight Time as we journeyed west on I-40 we arrived in mid to late afternoon. There are eight different housing locations that one could be assigned to at the Glade and this time we had a two-bedroom condo in Sterling Forest. Sterling Forest is in easy walking distance from the on-site shopping plaza, so after getting unpacked we walked to the grocery store. We didn't get too many items since we had to carry them back, and further, we would be walking the trails during the week and could pick up items anytime we were out. I played golf on three of the four courses they have at the Glade, did a puzzle, and read two books. Muriel, of course, buzzed through several of her pile of books. I walked the trails in the morning for exercise when I wasn't playing golf, and in the afternoon Muriel and I took walking excursions. We drove into Crossville one day and checked out the stores in the shopping mall. As many times as we had been to the Glade we had never taken the time to drive into Crossville.

On the following Friday we packed up early and headed west on I-40 on our way to Amarillo, Texas. We passed through Amarillo, left I-40 at Clines Corners in New Mexico, and drove north toward Pagosa Springs in Colorado. As we climbed up through the southern Rockies the temperature dropped significantly from that of Tennessee. By the time we got to Pagosa Springs we had passed into another time zone. It was dark when we checked in. We stayed in the B half of a split condo in Peregrine Village. During the three weeks we were in Pagosa Springs I drove to Wolf Creek six different times to ski. I completed the other two puzzles and the books I brought. Since Muriel had brought along several books I began to read some of the books she had finished.

The time we were away was meant to be a time to recoup and assess where we were and where we might possibly be going. Muriel was amazingly upbeat and was still looking forward to reaching our 50th wedding anniversary. My attitude was and still is that as long as she was positive I would be totally supportive, and if she faltered I would still be positive. One of the main reasons that we are on this trip is her desire to have me lead what she terms a "normal life." She has always been greatly concerned that I spend too much time in caring for her and carting her around to all of the doctor's appointments, scans, and blood tests. She is hopeful that Dr. Cline, after the colonoscopy, will be able to make a diagnosis that will eliminate the diarrhea. I judged that the time away was good for us both, and we were looking forward to returning and soon to be heading into a new year.

We left on Friday the 7th of December, the day, as Franklin Roosevelt said, "which will live in infamy." However, as we get further away from that date in 1941, we hear less and less about it. Perhaps it is a reflection of our age. We probably could have driven the trip in two days, but we allowed ourselves three and arrived home yesterday on the 9th.

Wednesday, December 12, 2001

Over the first two days that we were back, we had taken care of our mail, picked up the newspapers, and done the dirty laundry. Today we were back to formally taking care of Muriel. We had a scheduled visit to see Dr. Koenig and then for Muriel to have an Aredia treatment. She was weighed (121¼ pounds) and had her blood pressure taken (110/80). Dr. Koenig, of course, asked about the diarrhea and unfortunately got the same answer that he has gotten for eight months. Other than that her only other concern was the fact that she does not seem to have much of an appetite.

We left the examination room for the chemotherapy room and found a free chair. After almost five weeks of not having a needle stick, Muriel was once again sitting there with her eyes closed and me holding her hand while Beth Stein found a spot on her left hand. She was thankful that it was Beth. I had brought the Phase 10 cards and we played while the infusion of Aredia was taking place. We finished a game prior to the completion of the IV so we just cooled it until the needle was removed and then returned to our home.

Friday, December 14, 2001

Today was a doubleheader day. I had a colonoscopy scheduled for the afternoon and Muriel had a follow-up appointment with Dr. Doncals in the morning. It was cold this morning, so I dropped Muriel off at the door so she could go directly to the radiation therapy department and not get chilled on the way. I parked in the deck and caught up with her before she went in to see Dr. Doncals, who joined us soon after we were ushered into an examination room. Upon entry she said, "Tell me the status of your diarrhea."

"Little has changed, every third day," Muriel said dejectedly.

"The Questran didn't help?"

"The Questran gave me leg cramps. Nothing has helped except the Lomotil and Kadian."

"How was your visit to Dr. Cline?"

"He thought that the diarrhea might not be related to the radiation. I'm scheduled for a colonoscopy next week to help with his prognosis. He also told me to keep taking the Lomotil and Kadian, if necessary, to shut it down."

She completed a physical examination and made an appointment for Muriel at the beginning of April. We returned home, and after lunch Muriel accompanied me as I drove into Akron for my colonoscopy.

Sunday, December 16, 2001

We went to church this morning and celebrated Holy Communion together. Communion has always been a very important aspect of Muriel's life and when we are able to commune together it is a religious experience that draws us closer together. For years, as noted earlier, we flip-flopped the services to be able to commune on a weekly basis. It is my judgment that as the disease has progressed, this time together at the altar, sharing the body and blood of our Savior, has become an integral part of the peace she received from the Lord.

At about 4:00 we left for Sonja Pusch's house, as she was again hosting the Chorale Christmas party. I had made a pasta salad and tiramisu cake yesterday, which was our contribution to the potluck dinner. All of the members of the Chorale and their spouses were present, and we shared an enjoyable evening of food and fellowship.

Wednesday, December 19, 2001

We left home early this morning to drive to the hospital so Muriel could register for her colonoscopy. After registration we went to the endoscopy department where she was soon called in and assigned a cubicle containing a bed and a stand. She was asked to strip and put on a hospital gown. It was indicated that she would return to the same location after the completion of the procedure and could leave her clothes. I took her glasses with me and left to return to the waiting room. I was informed by Dr. Cline that everything went well when the procedure was complete.

I followed Dr. Cline back to the cubicle where Muriel lay, still a little groggy. He pulled the curtain and departed. She was soon alert and I supplied her with her glasses and she proceeded to get dressed. The nurse on duty insisted that she be discharged in a wheelchair, so she waited for a volunteer to come and wheel her out the main entrance. In the meantime, I went and got the car and was waiting by the entrance when the volunteer brought her out.

Monday, December 24, 2001

The Chorale sang four numbers at the Christmas Eve candlelight service with Muriel directing. We went to Communion and got many nods and smiles as we came up the aisle hand in hand. We returned home for our usual Christmas Eve exchange ritual. We had the shrimp, the beef log, cheese ball, other cheeses and two different kinds of crackers, plus we had some rosé wine. We didn't dwell on it at all, but the question that hangs in the air is *Will this be our last Christmas together?* From Muriel's point of view we will be spending many more Christmases together. She has such a wonderful attitude, and it rubs off on everyone she is in contact with, especially me. We are ready, and look forward to the coming new year.

Wednesday, January 2, 2002

We spent a quiet New Year's Eve as well as New Year's Day, but that doesn't continue today as we had a 10:00 a.m. appointment with Dr. Cline. We go with great expectation that the colonoscopy will have discovered some malfunction in the evacuation system that will mean that maybe the diarrhea can be overcome. Five of the office's eight chairs were occupied when we came in. Digestive Health Consultants is a six-doctor practice, so there were bound to be several patients as more than one doctor was probably holding office hours this day. I accompanied Muriel into the doctor's office. Dr. Cline shared with us the results of the colonoscopy. He said it showed there was no indication of any problem in the bowel. He suggested two things to see if there was any answer to why Muriel was continuing to have diarrhea problems. The first was to have a 72-hour fecal fat count test, which meant collecting fecal matter in containers and then having it analyzed. The second was to have a small bowel fluoroscopy. He was inclined to go with the first procedure and then, if that test did not prove anything definitive, we could go for the second. In the meantime he suggested that she continue to treat the diarrhea in the same manner she had been, by using the Kadian and Lomotil. We left the office disappointed that the colonoscopy had provided no definitive picture of Muriel's malady, but accepting of a new avenue of search. I took Muriel home and drove into City Hospital to pick up the necessary containers for the 72-hour fecal fat test.

Thursday, January 3, 2002

Even though we went to an appointment this morning that had been scheduled three months ago, it always amazes me that we have often had doctor's appointments on consecutive days during this adventure. We drove to Kent to see Dr. Abood for Muriel's regular three-month follow-up. I dropped her off at the front door and then parked the car. She had already taken the elevator to the second floor and was in the doctor's office when I arrived. Dottie took us to an examination room where she collected all of the vital statistics: weight (120 pounds), blood pressure (122/70), temperature (97.8°), and pulse (80). She asked Muriel about her pain level and it was concluded to be a zero. Dr. Abood indicated that he had gotten a report from Dr. Cline regarding the colonoscopy, and Muriel informed him that she was beginning a 72-hour fecal fat test. She also indicated that Dr. Cline suggested she continue the regimen of Kadian and Lomotil to keep the diarrhea in check. He performed a physical examination and also commented on the fact that her weight was down eight pounds from the previous visit. He checked on her breathing and asked how all the puffers were working for her. Muriel provided a satisfactory answer and asked for renewals for two of them. He also gave her an order for blood work that she will have to do another day because fasting was necessary. We left with an appointment in another three months.

I got Muriel squared away in her La-Z-Boy in the family room and I departed to go skiing. I drove her car so I could stop and get gas on my way home. There were a goodly number of skiers, but the lift lines were not long at all and we spaced ourselves well. I left when the buses came to disgorge hordes of school children.

Saturday, January 5, 2001

I was up early to do my exercises, and then after breakfast I took all of the containers containing fecal matter to the lab at City Hospital. Can you imagine storing containers of fecal matter in the refrigerator? You do what you have to do to try and get answers to problems.

Tuesday, January 8, 2002

Back to the Aredia routine this morning. We had a 9:45 appointment, and we were almost immediately ushered into the pre-examination area. Muriel weighed 117½ pounds, another slight loss from the last time we were here. We were then led into the examination room for a check on her blood pressure (164/86). When Dr. Koenig came in, Muriel reported that she was still having diarrhea problems, that the colonoscopy showed nothing, and that she had just completed the 72-hour fecal fat test but had no results on that as of today. She also indicated that she was scheduled for a small bowel study on the 28th of the month. She requested a prescription for Levaquin as she judged she had an upper respiratory tract infection. He gave her a physical examination, provided two prescriptions, and we were on our way to the chemotherapy room.

We were fortunate enough to get the chair in the alcove this morning, and Muriel was the recipient of Beth Stein's needle work with an IV planted firmly in the left hand. We played Phase 10 while the Aredia was infused into her body. Usually when we play Phase 10 I do all of the shuffling and dealing of the cards as Muriel has to keep her left hand flat on the arm of the chair. I am also required to look away as she sorts her cards, which are face up, and arranges them, and then puts the arranged cards into her left hand. Then she is in a position to draw and discard with her right hand and play begins. This morning she got to Phase 5 before I had gotten past Phase 2 and easily won the game. After beating me we both read until the infusion was complete.

Saturday, January 12, 2002

We packed the car and began our drive for a week in Bayse, Virginia. I hoped to ski and Muriel was going to read and relax. We stopped at McDonald's off I-76 and had breakfast. We took turns driving as we usually do, and Muriel was driving as we got off I-81 in Virginia. As she came up the ramp on a right-hand turn she appeared to be ready to run into a line of reflector markers. I reached over and grabbed the wheel and pulled the car back onto the off-ramp. At the same time I shouted "Muriel!" With the sudden lurch of the car and my shout she was immediately back in control and brought the car to a halt at the bottom of the ramp. "Wow, I'm sorry. I guess I wasn't concentrating on what I was doing."

I tried to make light of it and said, "It's my job to admire the scenery and yours to drive," and gave a little laugh.

She seemed a bit embarrassed. "I think you should probably take over the driving."

We switched and I said, "I'm sorry I grabbed the wheel, but it looked like you were going to wipe out the whole line of reflectors."

"I probably would have."

Considering the winding road to the resort Muriel seemed happy that I was driving and we arrived without any further incident.

Saturday, January 19, 2002

We had a lovely week in Virginia. I skied five of the mornings and we, after bundling up, took short walks in the afternoon. At least this time around Muriel was able to step up on the curbs without any pain in the pelvic area. I did all of the cooking for the week, I completed another jigsaw puzzle, and we both read several books. We did talk a little bit about the driving incident and Muriel judged she lost her concentration for a brief moment. We let it go at that and I anticipated that we would again share the driving on the way home.

This morning we packed up and headed back to Ohio. I took the first leg of the trip and drove all the way to Breezewood, where we stopped for breakfast. After we had eaten Muriel began driving. She negotiated the tricky entry back on to the Pennsylvania Turnpike where I-70 and I-76 merged. In that stretch we encountered a section where the road was under repair and we were confined to one lane each way. It was a short-term repair and there were no barriers between the two lanes, and at one point Muriel was driving in the oncoming lane. Perhaps she felt comfortable in that lane because normally both lanes would be going in the same direction, or perhaps she was having another lapse. This time I didn't yank the wheel but said in a calm, non-accusatory tone, "You need to return to the proper lane and when we come to the next rest area I want you to pull off and I will drive the rest of the way home."

She made no comment and stopped at the next rest area where we wordlessly switched drivers. There were many times I used to snooze while Muriel drove, but those days now appear to be gone. My mind is telling me the cancer is having a deleterious effect on her brain. Perhaps the statement about metastasis of bone, brain, lungs, and liver was now beginning to play out in another area of her body. We drove along in silence until I said, "I don't think you should drive the car again after we get home."

"I think that was just an isolated incident. I'll be okay once we are back in familiar territory."

"That is probably a good argument, but I can't allow you to drive and then get a call that you've been in an accident."

"How will I get to the meetings of the support group? And to our once-a-month luncheons?"

"No problem, I will be happy to drive you to the proper places and pick you up when they are over."

"As if you don't do enough for me already," she said sarcastically.

"How about the members in your support group, particularly Linda, Sue, or Robyn? Each one of them would probably be happy to come and pick you up and cart you around wherever you want to go."

"I wouldn't want to impose on them."

"I think they have felt quite useless in providing support for you through all the changes you have been experiencing and any one of them would jump at the chance to be of help."

"I'll try Robyn. She'd probably do it."

"I know this is difficult for you sweetheart, but I want you to promise me you won't drive after we get back home."

"What if I don't promise?"

"I will just have to get rid of your car right after we get home."

I think she knew that it would be better for her not to drive, and she ultimately promised me she wouldn't drive. I now have a new task to take care of, and that was to dispose of Muriel's car so that there will be no chance of her driving while I am out. However, she promised and that is good enough for me, so disposing of the car is not a priority.

Monday, January 28, 2002

This morning we went to City Hospital for a test on Muriel's small bowel. This was the test where one gets to drink that wonderful barium solution. Muriel was not looking forward to that. However, if doing so brought her closer to a solution for her diarrhea, then she was willing to continue the adventure. I went to see Karen Stewart, Dr. Koenig's business office manager, regarding a billing question and returned to the reception area before Muriel completed her test. She soon joined me and we left for home, stopping at Penney's on the way.

Wednesday, January 30, 2002

Today we celebrated our 43rd wedding anniversary. We shared the common card and speculated whether we would make it to our 50th. As far as Muriel is concerned, it is a done deal. She remains so positive, which helps me to be positive with her. Once again we enjoyed Duckling Rosé, wild rice, and asparagus. I had made a tiramisu cake the day before that we had for dessert. It was good to feel the closeness of our years together.

< 11 >
METASTASIS II AND MORE RADIATION

Wednesday, February 6, 2002

This morning we were back at Dr. Cline's office where we expected to hear the results of the small bowel test. He indicated that the small bowel was normal and he judged that Muriel has what is termed exocrine pancreatic insufficiency. Her body is not producing enough of an enzyme that allows for the digestion of fatty foods, so he prescribed Viokase. She is to take three tablets with meals and two tablets with snacks. In addition, he also provided a prescription for Protonix which was designed to reduce the acid in the stomach. It is assumed that the decrease in acid will aid the digestive system. This pill is to be taken daily. Maybe now we are on the right track to solve the problem of the diarrhea. I got Muriel back home, dropped off the prescriptions at CVS, and went skiing at Boston Mills through the lunch hour and early afternoon. I picked up the prescriptions on my way home and after I got back we went to the movies. From the movies we went to Applebee's for dinner.

Tuesday, February 12, 2002

This morning we went to Dr. Koenig's office for a check-up and for Muriel to have an Aredia treatment. Muriel was weighed (119½ pounds) and had her blood pressure taken (140/90). When Dr. Koenig entered the room he asked, "How was your visit to Dr. Cline?"

"The small bowel test didn't show anything, but he is treating me for exocrine pancreatic insufficiency and has put me on Viokase and Protonix."

"Have you seen any change?"

"It certainly has not stopped the diarrhea completely, but it appears to have lessened it. But then, it could just be me hoping it is better." She then shared about her driving experience to and from Virginia and that we had agreed that she should no longer be driving. She finished by saying, "I am having periodic aches in my back right along my spine."

He checked her medical record and said, "You should have a repeat of the CT scan for your chest and abdomen, as well as another bone scan. I also would like you to continue on the Arimidex and the monthly Aredia treatments." He then proceeded with a physical examination. When he was done we left to go to the chemotherapy room for Muriel's Aredia treatment.

Muriel had the chair directly in front of the alcove and I stayed with her while Beth Stein set up the IV. Radhika Mullins then took over and proceeded to draw blood to be tested. After the blood draw she set up the bag for the Aredia treatment. When Muriel was squared away I went back out to the scheduling clerk to make appointments for the CT scan and the bone scan, which were set up for this coming Friday and the following Thursday, respectively. I returned to the chemotherapy room and Muriel was busy reading, so I pulled up a stool and waited with her until the infiltration was complete. After she was free of the IV we walked to our car and headed out for lunch at the Applebee's at Chapel Hill Mall. After lunch we went to see the movie *Gosford Park* at the Plaza 8 at Chapel Hill.

Friday, February 15, 2002

For the first time in this adventure we were scheduled for the CT scan at St. Thomas Hospital. St. Thomas is part of Summa Health System and is located on North Main Street in Akron. It takes us just a little longer to get there than it would have taken going to City Hospital. I accompanied Muriel as she went to the room where the scan would be administered because I wanted to hold her hand when she had the IV set up. That accomplished, I returned to the waiting area while the test was administered. I was soon called back into the room and we departed for home.

Saturday, February 16, 2002

I have had a task on my "to do" list for the last couple of months and today I finally got around to doing it, and that was to dig out and read Muriel's long-term care policy. I have no idea when this disease is going to crop up next, but if she is going to be confined to an outside caring facility or confined at home I wanted to know what kind of coverage she has on her policy. I took the time to read through the policy and it looks like she is well-covered in either situation.

I washed sheets and made beds, and in the evening we went to E. J. Thomas Hall where the Akron Symphony Orchestra was playing a subscription concert. The program was all Mozart with Jaime Laredo as the conductor and who also served as the solo violinist on the final piece. The three Mozart pieces were Overture to *Die Zauberflöte*, K. 620, Symphony No. 5 in G Minor, K. 550, and Violin Concerto in E Minor, K. 216. There is always something about pieces by Mozart that tugs at your heartstrings and leaves you with a warm and fuzzy feeling.

Thursday, February 21, 2002

Today we had the second half of the scan doubleheader. This was the bone scan and requires a trip home after the first scan and then back to the hospital for a second scan. I stayed with Muriel while she had the IV put in and then retired to the waiting area while the technician administered the scan. I did some errands in between the trips to the hospital and when we came home after the rescan the day was gone.

Sunday, March 3, 2002

This past week we flew to Fort Lauderdale and then bused down to the dock area where we boarded the Royal Caribbean Cruise Lines ship, *Enchantment of the Seas*. We were on the western swing which included Haiti, Jamaica, Grand Cayman, and Mexico. Whenever we have cruised we have been content with an inside cabin, because the only time you are in the cabin is to sleep and it really wasn't necessary to be able to look out a porthole at night. We each brought several paperbacks with the idea that if you read all the ones you brought you could start on the ones the other person had brought. We did not take any of the excursions, but we did get off the ship at the ports where we were docked. We also tendered into Georgetown, Grand Cayman.

Cruising for us was not so much a sightseeing thing but an opportunity to relax and read, enjoy the great food and nightly shows, and soak up the sun. Muriel came fortified with her medications for the diarrhea as well as the reoccurring pain in her back. This was a trip with "casual dining," which meant there were no assigned tables and we could sit alone or with someone in the regular dining areas. Sometimes we just went to the buffet where all of the main dishes were being served as well and we liked the total informality. We arrived home yesterday, having returned to Fort Lauderdale before continuing home on the same day.

Monday, March 4, 2002

Today is my sister Karen's birthday. I had remembered to get a birthday card for her before we cruised, which I then mailed from Fort Lauderdale so she would get it on time. She is 61 and still working hard and loving it. It is also the day we are scheduled to see Dr. Cline for a follow-up visit regarding the Viokase/Protonix regimen. Muriel explained that there was no change with the diarrhea and was still taking the Kadian to shut it down. He was pleased that her weight had stabilized and he judged that the use of the Viokase and Protonix were contributory factors. He gave her a complete examination and suggested she return in two months.

On the way home I dropped off the prescription for Kadian and also requested a refill of Vicodin, another pain inhibitor, prescribed by Dr. Koenig. I picked them up later in the day. I also sent in our tax forms for federal, state, and local. I am due for a refund so the whole idea is to get it in and enjoy the refund. We also did the last-minute packing as we are leaving tomorrow for Texas and then on to Colorado and New Mexico.

Sunday, March 24, 2002

On March 5 we embarked on yet another trip to Texas to visit our children and grandchildren. I did all of the driving, which Muriel was not happy about. However, ever since the trip to Virginia I have played chauffeur and there have been no problems. In addition, Muriel did get in touch with members of her support group and they have taken turns picking her up and dropping her off for each of the sessions they have had. We stopped for breakfast at McDonald's in Mansfield, our usual stop on I-71 heading south to Texas. We also had the same meal, sausage biscuit with egg and coffee. This morning I added an orange juice as I needed to take my morning pills. With our tummies filled we continued south and picked up I-70 west. We made periodic stops to walk around and use the restrooms and finally exited the highway for the night in Joplin, Missouri.

I also transported my skis as we were to join Kay and her family on a spring ski trip to Angel Fire in New Mexico the following week. In the morning we drove west a short way into Oklahoma and then dropped directly south on Route 69 heading for Texas. We drove directly to Muriel's sister's house in Arlington, Texas to spend some time with her and her husband. Judith is on dialysis and it is unlikely she will be able to travel if Muriel's disease worsens. She is on a nationwide listing for a kidney transplant, but because of her scleroderma her chances of receiving a transplant are very slim. Muriel and I had talked about the fact that her sister may die and that maybe she too would not be able to travel for her services.

Neither of them wanted to hang crepe, so we went out to dinner at a lovely Mexican restaurant, ordered dinner, had a pitcher of margaritas, and had a delightful time together. We stayed overnight and then spent the next day with them as well. They kidded about not seeing each other again but I think there was a certain tacit acknowledgment that this was probably the last time they would be together. From Arlington we went to Plano and checked into the Comfort Inn. That would be our headquarters for a few days.

We went over to Mark and Cathy's house in Flower Mound and got reacquainted with our youngest granddaughter, Emma. She is going on four and is into playing games. So I got the full treatment and the whole gamut of games that she had available. Fortunately I didn't get them all the first night. We went to a Chinese restaurant for dinner. It was a buffet and they had just about anything you could ask for. I loaded my plate with different kinds of chicken as well as some of the sashimi delicacies, and then I spotted this green stuff next to the sliced ginger root. I was informed it was wasabi. Okay, I thought, try something new. I put a large glob of it on my plate anticipating taking smaller dabs to put on my food. As I prepared my first mouthful, Cathy said, "You're taking too much Grandpa and you'll be sorry you did." I scoffed at the suggestion, but there was no question about it. I took too much and I definitely was sorry. I had to leave the table because I was so nauseous I thought I was going to throw up. The wave finally passed and I returned to the table. Needless to say I did not have any more wasabi that night. Everyone thought I got what I deserved since I heeded no one's warning. They were probably right.

Staying at the motel allowed us to have some control in our lives so we slept in and then enjoyed the fare at the Comfort Inn for breakfast. They had hot plates where you could make your own waffles. Those hot plates do a great job and I had two waffles for breakfast. There are so many shopping places along Preston Road that we spent the morning and most of the afternoon just checking out the variety of items that were available for purchase. We checked in with Kay to see when we would be departing on Saturday and then spent another evening with Mark and his family.

On Saturday morning we left for Angel Fire as a two-car caravan. Kay and Larry had rented a house and we arrived around sunset and got ourselves settled in by dusk. Muriel and I had our own bedroom, and as it turned out it was a good idea. We had been to Angel Fire on other occasions without any adverse effects for Muriel, however this time she really seemed to be affected by the altitude. She was a little lethargic the first evening and went to bed early to read. She was fast asleep when I came to bed. Prior to my going to bed we had agreed to be up early and standing in line for our lift tickets when the windows opened. Kaitlyn would stay and keep Oma company.

In the morning Kay, Larry, Kenton, and I went skiing. Kenton and I pretty much skied together. We had lunch on the backside of the mountain and agreed to wrap up our day by 2:30. We all met at the bottom of the lift and trekked to the car. When we walked in the door, Kaitlyn informed us that Muriel was sick and had thrown up. I was into the bedroom in a flash and checked on her. At the time she was sleeping. I did not want to let the mess sit there on the floor so I got a pan of water and a cloth and began the clean-up. She awakened while I was in the process and informed me that she felt very weak. I thought she was dehydrated, so I tried to get her to drink some water and to have some tomato soup with crackers. She seemed reluctant to eat but did have a little bit. She did eat more as the week progressed, but pretty much stayed close to the bed where she read and slept.

I think the disease and the altitude did a number on her, because when we got back to Dallas she seemed to be her old self. During the week at Angel Fire, Muriel, as she has done throughout her adventure, encouraged me to ski, insisting that she would be fine. I think she also realized that skiing for me was a renewing experience and that I would be in a better position to care for her if I could have those experiences. Back in Plano we returned to the Comfort Inn and spent additional time with both families during the week. We returned home on March 23rd.

Tuesday, March 26, 2002

We may have enjoyed our time away but we were quickly back to the reality of doctor visits, like today, when Muriel had an appointment with Dr. Koenig. We were to find out about the CT scan and the bone scan.

There was nearly another full house in the waiting room and we had a moment to relax before Muriel was called into the pre-examination room. She was weighed (117 pounds) and had her blood pressure taken (136/72). Dr. Koenig entered the examination room with the scans and proceeded to put them on a viewer.

He pointed out the little white spots on the scan and stated, "There appear to be new tumors on the vertebra and a further spread of the cancer. The tumors are in the area where you indicated you were having pain." Muriel was seated on the examination table and I was in a chair. Had we been close to each other I would have put my arm around her a little tighter. He continued, "I think you should have more radiation to see if those tumors can be killed."

"Will that stop the spread of the cancer?"

"Cancer is a metastatic disease and it cannot be stopped. Our best hope is to slow it down. Are you controlling the diarrhea?"

"At Dr. Cline's suggestion, I have been taking Kadian on a regular basis which seems to hold it in check. He also prescribed Viokase and Protonix for the diarrhea, but it seems to me that taking Kadian has been the biggest help in controlling it. I am also taking two to four Vicodin a day to control the pain in my back."

"The radiation should help to kill the tumors and reduce the pain you are experiencing. I'll set up an appointment with Dr. Doncals so we can get that started."

He then gave Muriel a thorough examination. Lastly he asked her to stop taking Arimidex, and instead prescribed Aromasin. He explained that taking Aromasin would provide adjuvant treatment after the surgery, radiation, and chemotherapy. So we left the examination room with a prescription, and an appointment with Dr. Doncals, the radiation oncologist, and walked across the hall to the chemotherapy room.

Muriel was able to get the chair in the alcove this morning and Karen Mascio successfully started an IV in her left arm. After the IV was set up and the line flushed, Radhika Mullins set up the Aredia drip. We settled in for our 90 minutes with a game of Phase 10. One game generally lasts close to 90 minutes, so we were done at approximately the same time as the drip was complete. I got Muriel home and prepared her some soup for lunch. She spent the rest of the day reading, dozing, and doing crossword puzzles in her La-Z-Boy. I also prepared dinner. We had a chicken stir fry with a lot of cut-up veggies. I made enough that we will get a couple more meals out of it.

Wednesday, March 27, 2002

Back-to-back days of driving into the physician's office center, this time to see Dr. Karlen, Muriel's gynecological oncologist. She was due to have a Pap smear. One wonders the need for such a test considering the extent to which the cancer has spread. However, Muriel was good about following a routine for the appropriate check-ups, so we were seeing Dr. Karlen today. After the test we came home via the Merriman Valley and went to lunch at Papa Joe's Restaurant. We each had a glass of wine and after our lunch arrived, I said, "You probably surmised what the scan results would be."

"No doubt about it," Muriel replied. "The pain has been similar to the first bone tumors I had in my pelvic area."

"In spite of what Dr. Koenig said, maybe more radiation will stop the cancer in its tracks."

"Don't I wish. However, I will keep praying for a miracle and do what I have to do to prolong my life. I want us to celebrate our 50th wedding anniversary."

"Should we ask Dr. Koenig if there is any program at the Cleveland Clinic or elsewhere in the country that you could become a part of?"

"No, I do not want any extraordinary measures taken to keep me alive. I do have one request and you already know what that is."

"Yes, I know, make sure you are pain-free."

"You have to promise me."

"You know I can't make an outright promise but I will do all in my power to see that it is true. Please know that I love you so much and would not want to see you unduly suffer." We finished our lunch and returned home.

Friday, March 29, 2002

As if Muriel has not had enough needle pricks lately, today I took her to Lab Care where she had a blood draw for a lipid panel. This was requested by Dr. Abood, who is monitoring her total cholesterol, HDL, LDL, and triglycerides. She is scheduled to see him next week, so getting blood drawn was anticipatory to that visit. This way he will have the results when she has her appointment.

Tuesday, April 2, 2002

We began the day with a trip to see Dr. Doncals, Muriel's radiation oncologist. She entered the examination room with the same scans that Dr. Koenig had used, and placed them on the light screen. She began, "As Dr. Koenig told you, all of the spots represent new tumors and in my discussion with him we agreed that you should have another round of radiation."

"I know, and I am prepared to go ahead with the radiation."

"It's not quite that simple Muriel. You need to fully understand the gravity of having more radiation. Most of the radiation would be applied at or near where you had the radiation the first time around back in March of '99. There could be some short-term effects such as tiredness, a skin reaction, dry cough, esophagitis symptoms, difficulty eating, weight loss, and low blood counts. In addition, there may be long-term effects resulting from the double shot radiation to the same area. Long-term effects may include spinal cord injury, nerve injury, esophageal injury, and lung scarring. I think you should take a moment and discuss it with Keith." She then left the room to give us the opportunity to discuss the issues.

Concerned, I said, "That's a horrendous list of possibilities for further damage to your body if you have the radiation."

"It's my body and I want to proceed, and the sooner the better."

"I guess that ends the discussion."

"Yes it does. I want to get rid of the pain and I'm sure radiation will do that, just like the last time."

Dr. Doncals returned shortly thereafter and Muriel said, "I would like to go ahead with the radiation, but I do have one question."

"Yes, go ahead."

"Will this remove the pain I am experiencing?"

"There are no guarantees but I believe that your experience will be similar to the last time you had radiation." She again talked briefly of the probabilities of additional consequences and then gave Muriel a thorough examination. When she was done, Muriel said, "We are scheduled to go to Myrtle Beach on the 20th of April. Do you see a problem with that?"

"No, we will schedule radiation prior to that and when you return you can complete the sequence." We left knowing that Muriel will undergo radiation every day for four weeks broken into two sequences.

Wednesday, April 3, 2002

Fortunately for Muriel there were no appointments on April Fools' Day or we might have thought there was a cruel force in action. However, since that day we have entered a phase where we are on the road, with the exception of weekends, for twelve straight days. Today we traveled to Kent to see Dr. Abood. It is the three-month follow-up and sometimes it is difficult to believe that three months have elapsed since the last time we visited. I let Muriel off at the door and parked the car. When I arrived in the office she was ready to be ushered into an examination room. Dottie took her vital statistics, recording her weight (119 pounds), blood pressure (118/70), temperature (98.7°), pulse (80), and respirations (14). Two minutes after Dottie left, Dr. Abood arrived. The initial conversation centered around the diarrhea. He had received Dr. Cline's memo and was aware that she was taking Viokase and Protonix, and further, that he had suggested the continued use of Kadian as the shutdown for the diarrhea. There was some brief talk of pancreatic insufficiency and having a hyperactive colon. Muriel shared with him the results of the bone and CT scans showing the new metastasis in the vertebra. She indicated that starting tomorrow she will be undergoing 20 rounds of radiation therapy. Next came a discussion regarding the use of the puffers Muriel is using and the benefits she is receiving. Muriel was very positive. He indicated that he had gotten the results of the lipid panel and that the numbers were good all around. Lastly he examined her thoroughly, wrote some 90-day prescriptions, and we were on our way home with an appointment in another three months.

Thursday, April 4, 2002

We drove to City Hospital this morning and we once again began the routine of dropping Muriel off at the door and I parking the car, getting the parking pass stamped, and joining Muriel as she waited to be called in for the radiation treatment. It will be the routine we will undertake for the next 11 days.

Thursday, April 11, 2002

After we returned from radiation therapy we had lunch and then called at the funeral home to pay our respects to Dorothy Garcia, the surviving spouse of Emil "Mel" Garcia. The Garcias were the second family to move to our street about a month after we had taken up residence, and occupied the home kitty-corner across the street from us. They had two children who were just a couple of years younger than our children so there was some byplay as they grew from kids into teenagers. Earlier in the week Mel had slipped after showering and had hit his head on the corner of a chest. He never recovered consciousness. He often mowed our lawn when we traveled and I sometimes cleared his driveway with my snow blower. We wished to express our sympathy at his passing to Dorothy and the family.

Wednesday, April 17, 2002

Over the months since Muriel has stopped driving, I have been checking blue book prices for the car. I mentioned this to Kay when we were in Texas and she expressed an interest in buying the car for Kaitlyn, who would soon turn 16. We agreed on a price, and today I picked her up at the airport as she had come to take possession of the car. She was also going to join us for a week in Myrtle Beach. We spent about an hour at the title bureau getting a new title in her name.

Friday, April 26, 2002

Last Friday we left early in the morning for Myrtle Beach in a two-car caravan. With stops it generally takes us 12 hours and we arrived at just about 5:00. We stayed at SeaWatch Plantation, part of Fairfield Communities, and were assigned a two-bedroom villa on the second floor, overlooking the pool area. We had a Walmart right up the road from us where Kay and I shopped for the staples we would need for the week. I played golf a few times which provided some time for Muriel and Kay to spend together. In the evening we all went walking on the beach. When Muriel is at the ocean she positively glows. I suspect if she had her druthers she would elect to be on the beach when she dies. But since we have no idea when that will be, she is happy to grab snatches of this nirvana. Kay departed for Texas yesterday and this morning we left for Ohio. Muriel was totally renewed and ready to return to doing whatever she had to do to sustain her life.

Monday, April 29, 2002

Fortunately we had the weekend to get back to our routines and this morning we return to the continuation of radiation therapy. Muriel had completed 11 sessions before we went to the ocean so she has 9 more to go. Once again Muriel has accommodated me by having the radiation scheduled in the afternoon so I could play golf in the morning. It also benefits her as she gets to sleep in, so it is a win-win situation.

Tuesday, April 30, 2002

Today we got to make two trips to the hospital. We began the morning by going to see Dr. Koenig for a regular appointment, and then to have an Aredia treatment. Muriel's weight is back to 120 pounds and her blood pressure is 122/72. Dr. Koenig came through the door and asked Muriel how she was doing. She answered, "The radiation has really helped in reducing the pain in my back and I'm not using the Vicodin as often. I still have eight more radiation sessions after the one today. Do you think they will reduce the pain even more?"

"I can't predict that, but I think you will get additional relief when you have completed the series. How is the diarrhea?"

"I'm controlling it with the Kadian. If I don't take that the cramps are horrendous. I am continuing to explore solutions to the diarrhea problem with Dr. Cline and Dr. Abood. I also seem to tire more easily and often fall asleep in my La-Z-Boy recliner."

"Considering all that you have been through, such effects are to be expected. Hopefully you'll continue to benefit from the remaining radiation sessions, and we'll continue the Aromasin and Aredia."

He completed a physical examination and then we returned home, had a light lunch, and at 1:15 returned so Muriel could have her Aredia treatment. Muriel occupied the second chair in from the door and Liz Foley placed the IV in her left forearm. She cringed, but the first needle stick was successful. Muriel didn't feel like playing cards today so we both read while the Aredia was administered. After 90 minutes the vein was flushed, the needle pulled, and we were on our way home. As we walked to the parking deck I asked, "Considering all of the needle sticks you have been getting lately and who knows how many more are ahead of you, have you thought about getting a port put in again?"

"You know I hate to have needles stuck into my body but I don't even want to think about having another port."

"I was just thinking of you sweetheart, and how we might be able to reduce your discomfort."

"I know and I love you for it, and as long as you are there to hold my hand I'll survive."

After two trips today Muriel was ready to relax. I made dinner and then we went to Chorale practice. It was a long day for her.

Saturday, May 4, 2002

Since the beginning of the month Muriel has had three more radiation treatments and is feeling less and less pain. She judges it is a good day if she does not have to take any Vicodin. After Muriel arose late, I washed the sheets and made both beds. We relaxed for the rest of the day and for dinner ate last night's leftovers. After dinner we went to the Akron Symphony Orchestra subscription concert. It was the final concert of the year and music director Ya-Hui Wang had chosen Barber's Symphony No. 1 in One Movement, Op. 9, as the opening piece. After intermission the Akron Symphony Chorus was featured in Carl Orff's *Carmina Burana*. The chorus did an exceptional job on the piece and received the just applause of the listeners.

Monday, May 6, 2002

Today was a hectic day for me. However, it was my choice. I went to my breakfast Bible class and then out to play golf with our usual Monday morning foursome. I rushed home, showered, had a muffin for lunch, and then we drove to Cuyahoga Falls to see Dr. Cline. It was a follow-up visit to check on Muriel's well-being from the time he had prescribed the Viokase and Protonix. He was pleased that her weight had stabilized, and pointed out that she had actually gained two pounds. Of course, the diarrhea was another subject that was discussed. His final word on that was if the Kadian is doing the job and controlling the diarrhea, then Muriel should stay on it indefinitely. He gave her a physical examination and we departed.

From Dr. Cline's office we then drove to Akron City Hospital where Muriel was scheduled for her 17th round of radiation therapy. Because the weather was beautiful and we were early, I parked the car and we walked over to the hospital hand in hand. I said, "I so admire the way you have maintained such a positive attitude on your adventure."

"You know why it is easy to be positive. Way back in September of '98 I prayed for peace and God gave me peace and continues to do so each day. That makes coping easy."

"It's hard to keep up with you but I'm doing my best. I haven't missed any appointments you have had and I am sometimes overwhelmed at your fortitude and spunkiness in the face of all you have gone through. And God only knows what is still to come."

She offered me a smile and said, "Thank you sweetheart. Did you ever think that God's peace comes to me through your steadiness and the fact that you are there for me every single day?"

"Hey stop, you will have me crying." We walked in silence the rest of the way, allowing me the chance to gather my tears, and my thoughts about what she had said. The simple answer to her question was no. I had never imagined it that way. All along I felt I had had the good fortune of sharing in the surplus of peace God had afforded Muriel. But her question made me reconsider this.

We arrived at the radiation therapy department. I got the parking ticket validated while Muriel changed into a hospital gown. She sat holding my hand for about 15 seconds before she was called in for her treatment. Following her treatment she met with the radiation oncologist. We returned home and both of us relaxed in our recliners watching one of Muriel's "feel good" movies.

I have to admit I didn't pay much attention to the movie as I was unable to stop thinking about how we both had handled this adventure, trying to piece together the role of God and faith in its unfolding. God had given Muriel peace, but He had answered my prayers as well, giving me the strength to be there for her whenever she needed me, and now when she needed me most.

I understand these are matters beyond answer, but my thoughts left me with the impression that God had been there all along. Some might say it was serendipitous, but I know He led us to meet each other so long ago, and then led us to realize that we had forged a special, loving bond on that very first date. He planted the seed that bore those early firm roots that now, all these years later, have sprouted a mighty tree that is this wonderful symbiosis Muriel and I share. We have in many ways never been stronger, and I can't see how, given the circumstances, that would be possible without His intervention. Our growth, as nourishing and sustaining partners and as a family, has never ceased, and long after this tree has passed, our grove will flourish, a beautiful creation of eternal life on Earth and in Heaven alike. I thanked God again for all of our blessings and asked for the continuing strength we will need to face the challenges ahead.

Friday, May 10, 2002

Muriel finished radiation therapy today, a day later than expected, because on Wednesday the radiation therapy department called and canceled her projected appointment. After therapy we went to Amber Tree Service and Landscaping to purchase Muriel's birthday present, albeit a month early. This was the same garden store where we had purchased holly plants that enhanced the appearance of our home. I had asked Muriel what she wanted for her birthday this year and she said she wanted a white lilac tree. So we picked out a tree that looked sturdy and ready to grow. We drove home and I immediately set out to plant the tree in the backyard. I dug a hole, removed the tree from its pot, and planted it in the ground. I added some fertilizer and we gave it a generous dose of water. I said a silent prayer that we will have a flower by the time Muriel's birthday arrives.

Monday, May 27, 2002

Over the time since radiation therapy ended, we settled back into our regular retirement mode. We prepared for our house cleaner who came once a month. With all of the doctor's appointments it didn't seem like we were around enough to get the place dirty, but it was nice to have someone else do the work. With no pain in her back, Muriel was more energized and once again assumed all of the tasks that she had done over the years, but cautiously spread them throughout the week and pressed me into action where needed. She didn't say anything, but I have the sense that she judges herself to be out of the woods and can continue on with her life. That's what having the peace of the Lord in your being can do for you.

Tuesday, May 28, 2002

The last blip on this month's calendar was a trip to Dr. Koenig's office for Muriel's follow-up and an Aredia treatment. Muriel was weighed (117 pounds) and had her blood pressure measured (140/80). Muriel expressed to Dr. Koenig that she is pain-free after the radiation and has not needed to take any Vicodin at all. However, she did request a new prescription for the Vicodin as she wanted to be prepared if the pain returned. She also requested a renewal of her Kadian so that she can continue to control the diarrhea. He did a physical examination and provided Muriel with two prescriptions, and we then moved to the chemotherapy room.

Muriel was very fortunate to grab the chair in the alcove and was attended to by Beth Stein, Muriel's favorite needle lady. No muss, no fuss, and the needle was in with hardly a prick felt. Since we were in the alcove today we decided to play Phase 10. We had not quite finished the game when the 90 minutes had elapsed, so I packed up the cards and the scoring sheet knowing we would finish the game when we got home.

After we arrived home I went to Don Joseph Toyota Motors, where I picked up a brand new Toyota Camry. We had purchased Muriel's car and for many years I had leased the car I drove. However, with Muriel's car no longer with us, I decided to purchase this car as I don't want to have our children saddled with a lease if something should happen to both of us. So we end the month with a brand new car.

< 12 >
THE NEXT FIVE MONTHS OF 2002

Friday, June 7, 2002

It was a special day for Muriel as she participated in the American Cancer Society Relay for Life. A team from our church was walking to make people aware of breast cancer and raise money at the same time. The official beginning of the festivities had all of the cancer survivors out on the track to make the first loop, and each of them wore a special T-shirt indicating that she was a survivor. Five of the people in her support group also walked with her. It was an emotional time for them all. Since its inception the group has already lost two of its members, and even though nothing was said I'm sure there were thoughts that Muriel will be the next. After the initial walk around was complete and we heard all of the speeches, I took Muriel out to dinner to honor her for her participation. We drove up to Chapel Hill and went to Rockne's. It seemed rather fitting as it was the place where we had lunch after finding out about Muriel's first metastasis. She is now about one month from her last radiation treatment and looking forward to the rest of her life.

Tuesday, June 11, 2002

It may be hard to believe, but today one cluster of flowers on the lilac bush reached maturity, so after I exercised I went out with a pair of scissors and snipped it off. I put it in a bud vase with water to greet Muriel when she came downstairs for her morning cup of coffee. I had also placed the traveling birthday card on her side of the kitchen table. I then set out to paint a bench that we had purchased at the Home Depot, one of those wrought iron benches with the wooden slats. I did this in the garage since we no longer had two cars in there. I painted it completely black and placed it on our front porch where it blends well with the white colonial house and the black shutters. It will be a wonderful resting place when Muriel wants to be outside but not in the direct sun. In a sense it became another birthday present.

Thursday, June 13, 2002

This morning we drove to City Hospital where Muriel had another follow-up appointment in the radiation therapy department. Dr. Demas was the physician on duty and he always gives off an aura that says "I want to see the patient and no one else" so I never even bother to accompany Muriel when she is called into the examination room. According to Muriel, he was happy that she is pain-free and he said she should continue to use the RadiaCare to soften her skin in the area where the radiation was applied.

We often take walks in the evening as Muriel is determined to build up her strength in anticipation of the fall hiking season. She wants to earn another medallion to affix to her hiking staff. She continues to be so positive and I rarely hear her complain openly. She might groan a bit when she has a severe twinge of pain, but never feels sorry for herself, and in the process she has become a symbol of triumph over adversity for many in our church and in her support group. It always seems to me she is looking for what she can do to make someone else's life a little brighter rather than worry about her own life.

Tuesday, June 25, 2002

After I exercised this morning we made a trip to Dr. Koenig's office where Muriel had a regular check-up and then her Aredia treatment. The waiting room had several empty chairs, so we found two together and waited to be called in to the examination room. We did not wait very long, and as usual she was weighed (119½ pounds) and then had her blood pressure taken (130/60). Muriel reported that she has been pain-free and enjoying herself. She did mention that she still has the diarrhea but it was under control with the use of Kadian. Dr. Koenig examined her and we moved over to the chemotherapy room.

Muriel was able to claim the alcove chair this morning and Beth Stein placed the needle in her left forearm with flawless technique. Blood was drawn for analysis prior to beginning the Aredia drip. We played Phase 10 again today and all was complete by noontime. After we got home and had lunch, I cut Muriel's hair. I am not as nervous doing it, and she seemed pleased with the results. I made sure I only snipped a little at a time, and often had her check with the hand mirror to see if everything was satisfactory.

Monday, July 1, 2002

We left midmorning on the 28th for Canandaigua Lake in New York State for my 50th high school reunion. I actually went to Brockport High School in Brockport, New York but the committee had planned the anniversary celebration for Canandaigua. We had made arrangements to stay at the Bristol Inn right on Canandaigua Lake. We arrived around 4:00 and checked into this very rustic inn, with our room overlooking the golf course. Several of my classmates were also staying at the inn. There was an informal dinner there for those of us who journeyed in from out of town. The last reunion I had attended was the 25th, yet I still recognize many of my classmates. It was nice getting reacquainted and trading stories.

On Saturday, several of us played golf in the morning and then in the afternoon the committee had contracted for a ferryboat that was to sail around the lake with only the members of our class and their spouses on board. It was a beautiful day and Muriel and I moved about the boat from group to group sharing stories and listening to others. In the evening we had a formal dinner with the requisite speeches. One of those speeches was given by one of the teachers we had as seniors, and he and his wife attended as guests of our class. It was really great to see him and renew an old acquaintance.

I played golf again on Sunday with some of the remnant of the weekend, and then we returned to Ohio. Muriel thought it was a little tiring, but enjoyed visiting with my friends. She caught up on her sleep as she nodded off in the car on the way home.

Tuesday, July 2, 2002

Muriel and I did all sorts of errands this morning. We went to Acme, GNC, Kmart, Target, and Bed Bath & Beyond in addition to dropping off our water bill. In the afternoon Muriel had an appointment with Dr. Abood. We were ushered into an examination room by Dottie, who took all of the vital signs: weight (117 pounds), blood pressure (142/72), temperature (98.3°), pulse (84), and respirations (16). As soon as Dottie was done Dr. Abood entered the examination room. "How was the radiation on your back?"

"The radiation was completed in early May and I have been pain-free ever since."

"That's great. How about the diarrhea?"

"As you know, Dr. Cline found nothing in all of the tests I had and he suggested I continue to take Kadian on a daily basis, and that's what I have been doing."

"How are your allergies and COPD?"

"I have had shortness of breath in the morning, but it improves as the day progresses. No allergies so far. Maybe it's the use of the puffers throughout the day that has helped."

He proceeded with a physical examination. As we were about to depart he said, "I would like to see you in another three months, but I must inform you that soon after that I'm moving my practice to Aurora. You are welcome to move with me, but if you chose not to move I'll be happy to forward your records to whichever doctor you will be seeing."

"Thanks for letting us know. We'll need to think about that and will let you know what we decide," Muriel replied.

On our drive home I asked Muriel, "What do you think of that last bit of news?"

"Just what I need. How long a drive would that be for us?"

"The drive to Aurora would be about 50 miles round-trip."

"I don't want us to have to drive that far. I guess I need to find another personal care physician."

"Don't worry about it sweetheart. I'll get you a list of doctors for you to choose from."

Friday, July 5, 2002

We spent a quiet Fourth of July and this morning we went out for breakfast. I had one of those Friendly's coupons that was good for a free Big Breakfast if you purchased another one. If you are a coupon clipper you can't resist that. Muriel rarely eats breakfast except when we go out, so she was up a little earlier to enjoy this treat. She brought her shopping list, so after breakfast we picked up groceries for the month.

Tuesday, July 23, 2002

From the time we had seen Dr. Abood early in the month, our lives were pretty routine. We went to Blossom Music Center for Cleveland Orchestra concerts a couple of times, I continued to work in the yard, Muriel began planning for the upcoming Chorale season, we ate out a couple of times, and I began compiling a list of doctors so Muriel can select a new personal care physician.

However, this morning it was back in the saddle again and another posting to Muriel's adventure. We are visiting Dr. Koenig's office for a follow-up as well as an Aredia treatment. As usual Muriel was weighed (120 pounds) and her blood pressure was taken (130/60). Dr. Koenig asked, "Are you having any problems?"

"I am experiencing some discomfort in my chest. Actually, it seems to circle the whole body but centered in my back."

"It has been three months since your last scans, so I would like you to repeat the bone scan, CT scan, as well as an MRI. Those scans will enable us to better decide on a course of action."

Before moving to the chemotherapy room, he gave Muriel a complete physical examination. A chair right next to the bookcase became free just as we entered the chemotherapy room. Muriel positioned herself in the chair and Beth Stein proceeded with the task of finding a vein. She was successful on her first try and placed the IV in Muriel's left wrist. The first order of business was drawing a vial of blood for testing, then there was a quick flush of the line and the Aredia. Once she was squared away, I returned to the scheduling clerk to make arrangements for all of Muriel's scans. It took nearly a half hour, but all were put on the calendar: CT and bone scans on the 8th and the MRI on the 20th. When I returned to the room I tried to tuck myself back between the bookcase and Muriel's chair, as we were right by the door. We both read, waiting for the 90-minute infiltration to be complete. As we walked to the car I said, "You have the CT and bone scans on the 8th and the MRI on the 20th."

"Thank you for taking care of the scheduling, and I will also rely on you to get me to the right place on the right date at the right time."

"It's a done deal, sweetheart."

If she was beginning to be beaten down by all of the appointments, scans, blood draws, and the meds, she gave no indication. *Let's move forward,* that is her attitude.

Saturday, July 27, 2002

Muriel and I have often discussed whether or not she wishes to seek extraordinary measures if the disease progresses. She is pretty adamant about not going to any extremes. Her only request to me time and again is to make sure that her pain is under control, which I continually assure her I will do. Today we took a slightly different tack, as I received a call from Dr. Art Stennet. He had been an assistant pastor in our church many years ago, but got out of the ministry and went back to school. He eventually got his PhD, and is a practicing psychologist dealing with family and couple relationships. His phone call was to inform me about Seasilver. He had heard great things about it through some of his patients, and had tried it for some of the maladies in his life and that of his wife. It is touted to be beneficial for persons with any conditions, and he wanted me to be aware. He indicated that he had some literature and would send it to me if I liked. I thanked him for his concern and look forward to getting the information in the mail. I shared briefly with Muriel but she suggested we check out the literature Art was sending and then make a decision.

Monday, August 5, 2002

Early in the month the material on Seasilver arrived from Art Stennet, and Muriel and I read it thoroughly. She is willing to have me order some because even if it doesn't affect the cancer, perhaps it can stop the diarrhea. I placed an order for three bottles. We will make another decision when those are gone.

Thursday, August 8, 2002

Today was a very busy day for me, and almost as busy for Muriel. I awakened her very early as we had a 7:00 appointment at City Hospital for a CT scan followed immediately by a bone scan. We were over at St. Thomas Hospital for both exams, thank heavens for that. I sat with her while an IV was set up, and then retired to the waiting area. Things went pretty quickly and we moved to the bone scan. Fortunately for Muriel, at our request they left the IV in her arm so she wouldn't have to have a new one started for the bone scan. The bone scan, of course, is a double procedure with time in between. When the first scan was complete we left, and I took Muriel out to breakfast on our way home. We stopped at Bob Evans, where she had corned beef with two coddled eggs, whole wheat toast, and coffee. I settled for two eggs over easy, ham, whole wheat toast, and coffee. She really enjoyed the breakfast, as did I, as usually I have cereal for breakfast and generally she only has a cup of coffee and her pills. I suppose you could say we had a brunch, as it was going on 10:30 when we got home.

She was due back at the hospital by 1:00 and again was to drink lots of water. I took care of several items in preparation for our departure the next morning for Myrtle Beach. We were back to the hospital at 1:00 for the completion of the bone scan, then I brought Muriel home and hustled over to church where I got in on the last half of the bridge playing. After that it was back home to pick up Muriel to drive her to see Ann Bolf and get her haircut. She hadn't given up on me as a barber, it was just Muriel's way of helping out a friend, who was recently divorced, by becoming a customer for her hairdressing business. We were glad when the day was complete.

Friday, August 16, 2002

We have been going to North Myrtle Beach for the second week of August for many years, and on Friday the 9th we began the drive south one more time. Kay, Kaitlyn, and Kenton drove up from Texas to spend the week with us. By 9:00 in the morning Muriel, slathered in sun block, would be on the beach in her chair, watching the tide coming or going, observing people, or reading. Every now and again she would wade in the ocean or even swim a little bit, depending on how hot it might be. The ocean at this time of the year is always a pleasant temperature. At noontime she would come up to the condo to have some lunch and then head back down until approximately 4:00. The week at the beach is always very cathartic for her, and this week was no exception. If her mental attitude can conquer cancer, she is well on her way to success. Kay, Kenton, and I played golf a few times while Kaitlyn kept Oma company. In the evenings, we walked on the beach and then played UNO or Phase 10 and worked on the usual puzzle that I had brought. We ate in most of the time, as we had prepared three meals and Kay had prepared three meals. One evening we went to Barefoot Landing and ate at Damon's Grill, and then walked all around the shopping area. The week slipped by much too fast, and Kay and her family headed for Texas and we returned to Ohio.

Tuesday, August 20, 2002

Today we headed to City Hospital for an MRI. Both Muriel and I have had an MRI before, so she knew what to expect. While we waited for her to be called in, we talked a little bit about the claustrophobic effect. We both agreed that all you needed to do was close your eyes and pretend you were lying in bed. If you are lucky, you might even fall asleep. She was soon called in for the test, and just as quickly returned with the test complete.

In the afternoon I drove Muriel to an appointment with Dr. Beyer, her ophthalmologist. Her cataracts are stable and she does not need a change in her prescription.

Dr. Beyer said, "You're good for another year."

On the way home I asked, "How did you like the succinctness of that report?"

"That's the kind of report I need to get on a cancer check-up."

"Wouldn't that be great!"

Tuesday, August 27, 2002

Muriel had used the rest of the Seasilver, and judged that she had experienced little or no relief for her diarrhea. She also thinks that it will have no effect on the cancer, so the decision was made not to order any more.

Midmorning we were in Dr. Koenig's office for a follow-up visit, and then Muriel was to receive an Aredia treatment. She was weighed (115 pounds) and had her blood pressure taken (126/70). Dr. Koenig had a bounce in his step as he entered the room and reported, "The results of the scans indicate that cancer is present, but there is no evidence of anything new."

Muriel said, "The pain in my chest that I have previously experienced is gone and I am doing quite well. I did have diarrhea but the Kadian shut it down. I would appreciate a prescription for Levaquin. We are going to France on the 9th of September and I want to be prepared in case I experience a sinus infection."

"Just call next month, prior to leaving, and I'll have a prescription called in to the CVS in your area."

He completed a physical examination, and we then departed for the chemotherapy room. It is just a few steps from the examination room to the chemotherapy room where Muriel was able to take her favorite chair in the alcove. At this stage nearly all of the nurses accede to Beth Stein to find a vein and put in the needle. That's what happened this morning, and then Radhika Mullins took over and completed the IV. No blood draw this morning, so I dealt out the cards and we played Phase 10 while the drip went on. The infiltration was completed at 12:30 and we headed home.

Wednesday, September 4, 2002

I went to CVS this afternoon to pick up the prescription for Levaquin, which Muriel had requested from Dr. Koenig, in case it is needed during our trip to France.

Saturday, September 28, 2002

Our bags were packed, and on the 9th of September Art Tischler drove us to Cleveland Hopkins International Airport where we boarded a flight to JFK in New York. We were able to check our bags all the way to Nice, so we would just need to manage our carry-ons. We were in New York midafternoon and at 7:30 we boarded our overnight flight on

Northwest Airlines for Nice, France. We were picked up at the airport by our tour guide and driven to the Radisson Hotel located right on the Mediterranean, with a huge beach and boardwalk right across the street from our hotel. We spent a total of three days in Nice touring the area by bus and taking a day excursion to Monaco. We saw the Prince's Palace of Monaco and the grave of Princess Grace inside the cathedral. Some members of our group went to the Monte Carlo Casino, but we were content to just view it from the outside.

We traveled by bus to Aix-en-Provence, where we spent the day touring the city, and then on to Arles. On the way to Arles we stopped at the wooden drawbridge made famous in a painting by Van Gogh. We arrived in Arles in late afternoon and boarded the riverboat *MS Debussy* that was to be our home for the next several days. We took a walking tour of Arles and were able to observe the influence of the Romans, most notably an amphitheater which is a replica of the Coliseum in Rome. We left Arles in the late afternoon on the *MS Debussy,* and traveled on the Rhone River to the walled city of Avignon. We enjoyed a walking tour of the city the next day, and particularly enjoyed the Papal Palace. Our tour continued with stops in Viviers, Tournon, and eventually Lyon. In Lyon we observed an outstanding example of trompe l'oeil. We stood for several minutes mesmerized by the seeming reality of what we were looking at. We had a bus tour of Lyon with many stops to observe the historic spots of the city.

Our next stop was Macon where our ship docked on the Saône River and we debarked for a tour of the Clos de Vougeot vineyard and winery. The highlight was sampling the Pinot noir wine. We journeyed on to Beaune, where we were privileged to view the Hospices de Beaune. It is now a museum that depicts its past. In addition we enjoyed a walking tour of the city. We had signed up for the post-trip extension, so we debarked the ship and departed by bus for Blois. On the way we visited the Basilica in Vézelay and had lunch at a restaurant nearby. Muriel had an opportunity to take a taxi up the hill to the Basilica, but chose to walk. It was a mistake, and it turned out to be a very telling example of the progress of her COPD. We started up the hill at a reasonable pace, but soon slowed to a crawl and then to making stops as we progressed up the hill. By the time we got to the top we were about ten minutes behind everyone else, and the first thing we did was find a place for Muriel to sit so I could get her some water. She recovered quickly and we returned to the group and the tour.

We stayed at the Hotel Mercure in Blois and visited the Abbey of St. Gregory. We also took side trips to Château de Chenonceau and Château de Chambord, both with beautiful gardens. We bused to Chartres and visited the beautiful cathedral there, and then traveled into Paris. We were in Paris for three days and saw all of the standard tourist fare, i.e., the Eiffel Tower, Notre Dame Cathedral, the Champs-Élysées, and the Arc de Triomphe. We also had the opportunity to visit Versailles, the opulent palace of Louis XIV, and Giverny, the home of Claude Monet. In the latter place we walked in the gardens, over bridges where the ponds held the famous lily pads.

Outside of the hill climb in Vézelay, Muriel was magnificent. She did not tire, and participated in everything, including an evening out when we went to the Moulin Rouge for dinner and the show. After the show Muriel commented to several of the persons in our group that I had seen more bare breasts during the show than I had seen in the past three years. We had just a wonderful time, and returned home renewed and energized for whatever is to come.

Monday, September 30, 2002

I had a list of three different doctors from which Muriel was to choose a new personal care physician. She chose Dr. Michael Maggio, and I placed a call to his office to make an appointment for November the 4th. With consideration of the incident in Vézelay, I also called Dr. Kenneth Kretchmer, a pulmonary specialist, and made an appointment for November the 7th. We now add two new doctors to the mix.

Tuesday, October 1, 2002

This is another doubleheader day, as we drove to Kent to see Dr. Abood this morning for Muriel's three-month follow-up. This afternoon we will head downtown for a follow-up with Dr. Koenig and then an Aredia treatment.

This would be the last visit to Dr. Abood, as he will soon be moving his practice north to Aurora. Dottie took all of the vital statistics: weight (117 pounds), blood pressure (156/80), temperature (97.9°), pulse (80), and respirations (18). When Dr. Abood entered the examination room Muriel informed him, "I have selected Dr. Maggio as my new primary care physician and have an appointment to see him in November. I would like you to send my records to his office."

"Of course. We can take care of it when you leave."

"I have also selected a pulmonary specialist, Dr. Kretchmer, and have made an appointment to see him in November as well."

"That's probably a good idea considering the difficulties you have experienced."

Dr. Abood asked about her breathing, the diarrhea, and whether she had any pain at this time. He completed a physical examination. Lastly, he requested that she have a blood test. However, since it is a fasting blood test it will have to wait until tomorrow morning. We shook hands all around and then completed some paperwork that would allow him to transfer her records to Dr. Maggio. We left the office for the last time.

We drove home for lunch, and then got back into the car for a trip to the physician's office building and a date with Dr. Koenig. Apparently most of the cancer patients are seen in the morning, as the waiting area was rather sparse. We were quickly called into the pre-examination area where Muriel was weighed (117 pounds) and her blood pressure was taken (138/80). Much of the conversation centered around our recent trip to France, and outside of the incident in Vézelay Muriel indicated that she had no difficulties, no pain, and that the Kadian keeps the diarrhea in check. She thanked him for the prescription for the Levaquin, but she didn't have to use it. Next followed the usual physical examination. Before departing for her Aredia treatment, Muriel requested refills for Valium and Kadian. Since both of these are narcotics, we have to take them to CVS for a 30-day supply. Most of the other prescriptions she takes are received through mail order where she can get a 90-day supply, so we work within the system.

From the examination room we moved to the chemotherapy room. There were only two other persons in the room, so we had our pick of chairs. However, the alcove chair was occupied, so Muriel took the chair right in front of that one. Beth Stein once again administered the needle prick and set up the IV. Muriel was content to read today, so I sat on the stool at her side and read also. The 90 minutes passed by very quickly, and we returned home where I had the privilege of mowing the lawn. At one point I had gotten a lawn service to mow my lawn, because my philosophy was that if it was nice enough to mow the lawn it was nice enough to play golf. However, Muriel did not like the way they did it, so I was pressed back into action. I think she liked the pattern I used, changing direction of the mower each time I mowed.

Wednesday, October 2, 2002

I played golf in the morning and Muriel slept in. When she did get up she fasted, so she was ready to be taken to her blood test when I came home. We went to the outpatient laboratory of Robinson Memorial

Hospital in Kent, where a very gentle woman made an "imperceptible" stick, as Muriel described it, and withdrew blood. I was happy for her.

Thursday, October 3, 2002

We seem to be getting everything out of the way at the beginning of the month, as today we are on our way to the radiation therapy department for a follow-up. I dropped her off at the door because there was no need to have her walk extra steps. I caught up with her in the waiting room, where she had switched to a hospital gown and was waiting to be called in for examination. If one has to go for a check-up, regardless of what it is for, one should have the privilege of seeing someone like Dr. Doncals. Her pleasantness and interest in her patient is just outstanding. She first wanted to hear all about our trip to France, which Muriel related with limited detail. She then examined her, asked some questions, and then suggested we make an appointment for March of '03. On our way home we made several stops including GNC, where we picked up some supplements, and New Earth, where Muriel picked up some additional herbals.

Since we had been in France during much of September, we did not have an opportunity to begin our quest for another medallion during the Fall Hiking Spree. So we hiked trails on Friday, Saturday, and Sunday. One of them was a three, and Muriel really struggled with it, stopping many times to catch her breath. After that we made the decision to only complete eight trails, the minimum, and no more threes.

Sunday, October 27, 2002

For the week beginning October 7th, I was making reservations for a domestic jaunt starting in Williamsburg, Virginia, then to Charleston, South Carolina, Atlanta, Georgia, and finally on to Columbus, Ohio where we were to meet our son, Mark, and go to a couple of hockey games between my alma mater, Clarkson University, and the Ohio State Buckeye hockey team.

We packed the car and left for Williamsburg on the 12th. We drove across Pennsylvania to Breezewood, and then dropped south on I-70 into Maryland where we picked up I-270 into Frederick. Next came I-495 around DC, then I-95 south to Richmond, and finally east on I-64 to Williamsburg. We were booked into the Governor's Green, part of Fairfield communities, which became our base for the week. We have been to the historic village several times, but we are always fascinated with the period restorations. We had one evening meal at Chowning's Tavern, and had brought meals for the other nights. I played golf out at the Colonial Heritage Golf Club and we trekked through the Williamsburg Pottery Factory as well as Merchants Square.

On Saturday the 19th we drove into Newport News and then traveled local roads along the bottom of the state back to I-95. We stayed on that interstate until we reached I-26, which took us right into Charleston. We stayed at the Days Inn right in the historic district. Armed with our AAA tour guide, we did the walking tour of all the historic homes. It was the first time I had been exposed to the front door opening onto a porch or a piazza as it was termed, basically a false entrance. We were fortunate to be able to take a trip to Fort Sumter, and basked in the historical significance of the place.

On Tuesday the 22nd we packed up our things, returned to I-95, and drove northwest toward Columbia. Out of Columbia we took I-20 toward Atlanta. We arrived after lunch and checked into the Days Inn on Spring Street in downtown Atlanta. We visited Atlanta Underground that afternoon, and the next morning we toured the CNN studios. After lunch we headed north on I-75 and drove to Chattanooga and then on into Knoxville where we stayed overnight.

The next morning we continued our journey north to Columbus, Ohio. We met Mark at the motel we had booked, and went to dinner and then to the hockey game at Schottenstein Center on the campus of OSU. Unfortunately, Clarkson lost. We had anticipated spending Saturday in Columbus, as the two games were Friday evening and Sunday afternoon. However, I think all of the travel had taken a toll on Muriel and she wanted to go home. We expected that Mark would go with us, but he chose to stay at the motel and watch football Saturday afternoon. So Muriel and I went by ourselves, and she was very happy to be home. I returned on Sunday, picked up Mark, and we went to Bob Evans for brunch. We spent some time touring the Jack Nicklaus Golf Museum prior to the hockey game. After the game, which Clarkson also lost, I took Mark back to the motel and headed home.

Monday, October 28, 2002

This morning I took Muriel to the dentist, waited for her to have her teeth cleaned, and then we went to Walmart. I also picked up the mail, sorted through it, and took care of some bills. Since Muriel had all of the food out and a ready recipe, I made dinner this evening.

Tuesday, October 29, 2002

Four weeks have passed and it was time once again to see Dr. Koenig. Whenever we visit Dr. Koenig, I sometimes think that we are waiting for the other shoe to drop, but Muriel continues to be positive with little or no complaints about pain. There is definitely an acceptance of the diarrhea that is basically controlled through the use of Kadian. So we keep moving forward. She was weighed (113 pounds) and her blood pressure was taken (100/60). Muriel and Dr. Koenig chatted a bit regarding her condition, and he seemed satisfied that she was doing well. Next came the physical examination. With that completed, we moved to the chemotherapy room for another Aredia treatment.

Muriel was able to have the chair in the alcove this morning, and Beth Stein found a vein in her hand with no difficulty. I have never had a problem with having needles stuck into me, and generally watch while it is being done. Muriel, on the other hand, has never watched, and in fact doesn't even want the nurse to say when the needle is coming. Just get it done. With Beth, that is the way it has been. She just gets it done. No warning, and very little pain. Muriel has been thankful for that throughout this whole adventure. We played cards this morning and I was soundly beaten. When we returned home, we filled out our absentee ballots which had arrived in the mail, extending our voting record for another year.

Thursday, October 31, 2002

This morning I had to go to Dr. Koenig's office to pick up a prescription for Kadian, which I dropped off at CVS on my way home. When I got home, I was the recipient of the common birthday card and a special hug and kiss for my 68th birthday. In honor of the occasion we had dinner at the Romano's Macaroni Grill out in Montrose. We really enjoy the fresh bread you can dip in olive oil with black pepper. I had the pork chop dish with penne pasta and a marinara sauce. Muriel had a shrimp dish with angel hair pasta, also with a marinara sauce. We both had a fresh garden salad. To accompany the meal, we each had a glass of house Merlot. For dessert we shared a piece of tiramisu cake. We had a good time and just enjoyed each other's company.

Saturday, November 2, 2002

Ever since I had open heart surgery, I have walked in the annual Heart Walk if I was in town. So today I donned my red hat and participated in this year's event. They have moved the walk from the Fairlawn area to the campus of the University of Akron, which makes the trip much shorter for me. It was well-organized, with the walkers gathering on the pavement outside the James A. Rhodes Arena and the registration inside in the lobby. Based on the check that I presented, I was given a bag of goodies that I put in my car so I wouldn't be burdened on the walk. I was back home by noontime. Although Muriel is getting good reviews from Dr. Koenig, I see her tiring more and resting whenever she has the opportunity. She has always been one to sleep in whenever she got the chance, but lately she is happy to stay in bed until noontime. With her resting, I made dinner this evening.

Monday, November 4, 2002

Today Muriel makes her first visit to Dr. Maggio, her third primary care physician during this adventure. I suppose the specialists are the important ones on this journey, but the primary care physician sees to the day-to-day maladies and helps keep the patient's life on an even keel. Muriel went armed with her usual list of medications, as well as a listing of all of her doctors. The nurse weighed her (114 pounds), measured her height (5' 2"), took her blood pressure (120/80), took her temperature (99°), and her pulse (80). Dr. Maggio, a very personable individual, greeted us and indicated that he desired to care for Muriel's well-being in the best way possible. Through questions and answers, he found out all about the cancer and what is happening at the present time. Muriel told him of the COPD and that she has an appointment with Dr. Kretchmer later in the week. In discussing the COPD, Muriel told him that currently she has a cough, draining mucous from her nose, and had a temperature of 100° earlier in the morning. She judges she had a sinus infection, a malady she is prone to get periodically.

He gave her a physical examination and also two prescriptions, one for doxycycline and another for an Atrovent inhaler which she has used in the past. He also wanted her to have a chest X-ray and provided us with an order to get it done.

We left the office and drove further up Route 91 toward Hudson, where there is an outpatient facility that does chest X-rays. On the drive up Muriel commented, "I surely have been blessed with good, caring primary care physicians, starting with Dr. Marshall back in Potsdam, and I judge Dr. Maggio can be added to the list."

"You mention Dr. Marshall. Wow, that was a long time ago."

"I didn't want to leave anyone out, and he was the first."

We were quickly in and out of the X-ray facility and on our way home. I dropped off the two prescriptions at CVS, which was on the way, and then picked them up later in the day. After we returned home, Muriel got all the ingredients together for dinner. I suggested she cool it, and I made dinner.

< 13 >
CHRONIC OBSTRUCTIVE
PULMONARY DISEASE

Thursday, November 7, 2002

This morning a new doctor entered the picture as we left home to see Dr. Kretchmer, a partner with Akron Pulmonary Associates, Inc. Since it was our first visit, it was necessary to go through all of the history and get the doctor and the office up to speed on Muriel's medical status. She was given a respiratory examination that included the vital statistics of weight (115 pounds), pulse (105), blood pressure (144/78), temperature (97.4°), and oxygen saturation (80%). He did a physical examination relative to her COPD. When all was complete he prescribed continuous oxygen at three liters per minute, increased the Advair to four puffs four times per day, and gave her a prescription for prednisone. Lastly, she is to return in two weeks to see how things are going. I don't think Muriel likes the idea of going on oxygen full-time, but she quickly resolved it in her mind as the best thing for her quality of life. We dropped off the prescription on the way home and I picked it up later. When we got home, I called Fairfield Glade to cancel the week we had scheduled beginning on Friday. I cooked our dinner tonight.

Thursday, November 14, 2002

Muriel was pretty much back to normal as the week began. We even went to the movies on Tuesday, as we wanted to be out of the house when the cleaners came. On Wednesday we hiked the trail in Gorge Metro Park. Needless to say we took a lot longer than we have in the past, but Muriel is determined to earn her medallion for 2002. That hike completed the minimum number of trails, so when I turn in our hiking sheets we will receive another medallion. Today we met with a respiratory specialist from Lincare who came to make an assessment of Muriel's condition and set her up for regular oxygen therapy.

Apparently 42 years of smoking has finally taken its toll. Muriel had quit in 1997, but the damage had already been done by that time. I had quit smoking in 1989 and I, her children, and her grandchildren had asked her to stop. I think she stopped for each one of those constituencies at different times over the years, but it never lasted because she didn't quit for herself. However, she went out of the way to accommodate me, as she never smoked in the car after I quit and always smoked in the garage when she was home. Some of those cold winters were pretty tough. What it did accomplish was a great reduction in the number of cigarettes she smoked per day. However, when she retired in 1997 she did quit, and often says to me that maybe if she hadn't stopped smoking she never would have gotten cancer. That, of course, is problematic.

After the respiratory specialist had completed the interview, we were supplied with an O_2 concentrator and 40 feet of tubing attached to a nose cannula that would allow Muriel to go anywhere in the house and remain on oxygen. We also received a container of liquid oxygen, which will be housed in the garage, and an Escort, a portable device that can be filled directly from the liquid oxygen container. I also received instructions on how to fill the container. The portable unit, when filled, will allow Muriel to be out for five hours on intermittent flow or about three hours on continuous flow. She will generally operate the unit on intermittent flow.

Perhaps it is important to picture our house as you think about Muriel moving around uninhibited yet attached to this 40-foot tether. As you enter the house from the front porch, there is a very small entryway. On the left is a closet for coats and hats. Moving directly ahead takes you up the stairs to the second floor. Moving to the right takes one into the living room and toward the formal dining area, which shares the same room. There is a door into the kitchen by the dining area and through the kitchen is the family room. In the kitchen there are three doors on the wall to the front of the house. One leads to the garage, one to the basement, and the other to a small half bath.

The family room has a fireplace on the back wall with bookcases on either side of it. On the left of the fireplace is a specially-built shelving unit that contains all of the video tapes that Muriel has accumulated. The room also has two La-Z-Boy recliners in front of the fireplace facing the television, a large 27-inch console. In the middle of the wall that faces the backyard are sliding doors that open onto a wooden deck. A sofa occupies the opposite wall with a coffee table directly in front of it. There are matching maple end tables at each end of the sofa that hold matching early American lamps. A lamp table is situated next to the other recliner. There are two symmetrically-spaced lithographs above the couch, and pictures of our children and grandchildren on the opposite wall closer to the kitchen. There is a half wall between the kitchen and the family room, with spindles from the half wall to the ceiling providing an airy atmosphere. The kitchen contains a drop-leaf table with two chairs and the usual appliances. Cabinets adorn the wall facing the backyard and straddle the window that is located above the sink.

The dining room contains a table with four chairs, and two more are on the back wall on either side of the window. There is a china cabinet against the outside wall and a credenza on the opposite wall. In the living room there are three matching pieces of furniture: a couch on the closed wall, a loveseat between the two front windows, and a chair just in front of a piano. There are matching end tables bracketing the love seat, with a drum lamp on each. The piano is located against the wall that leads to the upstairs. A floor lamp is located behind the single chair and also serves the piano. There are three other items in the room: a stand that supports the unabridged English Oxford Dictionary, a low cabinet-type table at the end of the couch, and tucked into the corner of the room is an easel that holds a needlepoint done by my mother. There are also five lithographs hanging on walls around the room.

There is a small space next to the piano and it is to become the home of the oxygen concentrator. The tubing is long enough to move any-where in the house, even to the basement. However, when going from downstairs to upstairs it will be necessary to move the tubing over the lamp and chair, or the lamp might be pulled over.

At the top of the stairs, a turn to the right takes you to two different bedrooms, one to the front of the house and the other to the back. The front bedroom is mine and contains a bed between the two windows, with matching end tables, a "university" chair, given to me by my colleagues when I retired, and two bureaus. The wall by the stairway is occupied by a floor-to-ceiling bookcase. On the opposite wall there is a built-in closet with folding doors. On the end wall of the closet there are more bookcases affixed to the wall. The other bedroom contains twin beds, a small storage closet, and more bookcases. A floor-to-ceiling bookcase is against the wall to the left as you enter the room, and there are bookcases on the wall opposite and on the right side that are attached to the wall from eye level to the ceiling. Lastly there is a desk below the window to the backyard and a bookcase to its right made with bricks and planks. On the wall above the makeshift bookcase is a display case holding Muriel's collection of miniature vases.

Coming up the stairs, to the immediate left is a full bathroom and then Muriel's bedroom, both facing the front of the house. The bathroom can also be entered from Muriel's room. Between the two doors is another freestanding waist-high bookcase. In the middle of the room on the opposite wall is a king-sized waterbed. There are two windows facing the front of the house with a desk beneath the right window. Next to the desk is a freestanding floor-to-ceiling bookcase. On the opposite wall is a built-in closet with folding doors, and on the closed end is a dresser.

The fourth bedroom is the smallest and contains two large open cabinets that house our computers. A printer is located directly under the window and another floor-to-ceiling bookcase is on the back wall with a built-in closet next to it. It is within the confines of these venues that Muriel will maneuver with her tether.

Saturday, November 16, 2002

It took but a few days before Muriel was fully acclimated to moving freely with tubing trailing behind her. Sometimes she will coil it up and other times she will just drag it wherever she goes. She probably can leave it off when she showers, but Muriel follows orders, so she removes the cannula, throws it over the partition, and puts it back on when she gets into the shower. We have sliding doors on our shower, and she does not want to pinch the tubing when closing the door. As she has done throughout this adventure, she quickly adjusted to the circumstances and is moving on.

This evening Muriel had her first opportunity to utilize her portable oxygen apparatus. It is designed to be worn on a belt that can be strapped around the waist. However, she vetoed that right from the start, and put the whole thing into a canvas shopping bag and carried it quite comfortably in her hand. We had tickets for Mandy Patinkin, who was giving a one-man show at E. J. Thomas Hall. When the portable unit was set to intermittent flow, there is a slight hiss on every exhale, and I was concerned that the patrons around us would be annoyed with this constant disturbance. Either it was not annoying or those seated near us were kind enough not to say anything. I think the one trip out on the portable oxygen convinced Muriel she can go anywhere. However, she was much like Cinderella, in that her time to be out was limited. We made it through the evening without a close call.

Thursday, November 21, 2002

This morning we had a follow-up visit with Dr. Kretchmer. I parked on the second floor in the deck and told Muriel, "Stay in the car until I get a wheelchair."

"I can walk to Dr. Kretchmer's office, it's not that far."

"Please, just stay in the car. There is no sense in taxing yourself when you can sit and be comfortable and let me do the work."

Since Dr. Kretchmer is located on the first floor, we took the elevator down from the second and I wheeled her into suite 104. She told Dr. Kretchmer, "I'm doing much better on the extra puffs of the Advair, and I judge that being on oxygen 24 hours a day has been very helpful." Her vital signs for the day were as follows: weight (114½ pounds), pulse (117), blood pressure (186/96), temperature (96.6°). She had her finger put into the little clip for the SpO2 reading, which measures the amount of oxygen expressed as a percentage being carried by the red blood cells in the blood. Initially it was 84% but after she sat awhile went up to 94%. Since 96% is normal, being on oxygen appears to be beneficial. Dr. Kretchmer seemed to be pleased with her improvement. "I want you to continue on the prednisone but begin to taper off, and since your breathing is better, I want you to continue on the Advair and Atrovent as well as continuous home oxygen." He proceeded to examine Muriel, listening through his stethoscope and inspecting her throat. After about 15 minutes we were on our way back home.

Friday, November 22, 2002

After lunch, I took Muriel to get a flu shot in Dr. Maggio's office. It was administered by his nurse, and we never did see Dr. Maggio. In the evening I filled up Muriel's portable oxygen tank and we went to see Ohio Ballet.

Wednesday, November 27, 2002

Today was a preparation day for Thanksgiving. We are going to spend the day at home, just the two of us. My contribution was the making of two pies, one pumpkin and the other butterscotch pudding. We always pack the latter with lots of walnuts. I also got out the food grinder and made cranberry relish. Muriel prepared the turkey and stuffing. In the evening, we went to church to celebrate our thankfulness for what God has done in our lives. The Chorale did several numbers during the service. We went to Communion together and reveled in the closeness we felt. Muriel received an undue amount of "atta-girls" from members of the Chorale and the congregation. We returned home with a closeness that I enhanced with the lighting of a fire in the fireplace. We watched a "feel good" movie, *An Affair to Remember,* as we abandoned our duo recliners and curled up together on the couch. As many times as I have seen that movie, I always cry at the end when Cary Grant discovers his painting in Deborah Kerr's side room. Tonight was no exception.

Thursday, November 28, 2002

Muriel slept in this morning and I did my usual exercise routine. I watched the Turkey Day parades while waiting for Muriel to make her appearance. She finally arrived on the scene about 12:30. I sought out instruction as to what I could do to help with dinner. I watched football in the afternoon and carried out the completion of the tasks I had been given for dinner. We ate in the dining room and really enjoyed the meal. Neither of us speculated about what the future might hold regarding her cancer. It is generally a specious subject, as Muriel's positive attitude always prevails. I cleaned up after dinner and cut up and packaged the leftover turkey, which went into our freezer for consumption at a later date.

< 14 >
DIAGNOSIS: THREE TO SIX MONTHS

Tuesday, December 3, 2002

Another doubleheader day. We began this morning by going to see Dr. Maggio. It essentially was the two-month check-up that Dr. Abood suggested the last time we saw him. Any movement for Muriel is getting to be more difficult because of the breathing problems she is experiencing. I dropped her as close to the door as I could, parked the car, and quickly caught up with her. The cold weather did not help at all. We hung up our winter coats and the nurse took us into an examination room. The nurse took her blood pressure (170/88) and Muriel's chief complaint was increased shortness of breath. When Dr. Maggio walked into the room he asked, "What can I do for you today?"

"I guess it's pretty obvious that I am now on oxygen full-time," she said.

"The cannula is a dead giveaway," he replied.

"I guess so, and I also have an oxygen concentrator at home that provides four liters of oxygen per hour. But right now I am draining a thick white and yellow mucous, and I also have a little bit of a cough, all of which are usually precursors for a sinus infection. I think I need a prescription for Levaquin."

"That's quite a litany of symptoms, but I think you should be on doxycycline instead."

"I judge for me that Levaquin is more effective."

"Let's take a look and then we can decide."

After completing his examination, he acceded to Muriel's wishes and provided her a prescription for Levaquin. We departed, and on our way home dropped the prescription at CVS.

After lunch we drove in the other direction for Muriel's appointment with Dr. Koenig and another Aredia treatment. I stopped at the hospital entrance, found a wheelchair, got Muriel into it, and then wheeled her inside to wait while I parked the car. I quickly returned and wheeled her to the Summit Oncology suite. She got out of the wheelchair to be weighed (117½ pounds) and then I wheeled her into the examination room where her blood pressure was taken (136/80). She told Dr. Koenig, "I saw Dr. Maggio this morning and he has put me on Levaquin for my sinus infection. Do you think this will prevent me from having an Aredia treatment today?"

"I don't think so, but let's do an examination to see if there is cause to delay."

The cannula at her nose prompted a brief discussion with Dr. Koenig about her use of oxygen. He then performed a physical examination and said, "There is nothing to prevent you from having an Aredia treatment today. However, I would like you to have another CT scan and a bone scan."

"I'll take care of scheduling that," I said.

Lastly Dr. Koenig wrote Muriel a new prescription for Kadian. Muriel's breathing problems together with the sinus infection were evident as she slumped in the wheelchair as I moved her to the chemotherapy room.

Because Muriel was in a wheelchair, she was placed in the overflow room. Radhika Mullins quickly found a usable vein in Muriel's left wrist and set up the IV. We were the only persons in the overflow room and Muriel was content to read. I used the time to make appointments for the CT scan and the bone scan. In a half hour I was back with the information and told Muriel, "Both scans are scheduled for the 11th of December."

"Thanks for taking care of that, sweetie." Muriel finished up the infusion and we headed home. We again stopped at CVS, picked up one Rx and dropped off another. In spite of the busy day and the tiredness she felt, after dinner we went to Chorale practice, which seemed to perk her up. The Chorale is due to sing at the first Advent service and she wants them to be prepared. We picked up the latest prescription on our way to practice, and upon our return Muriel went quickly to bed.

Wednesday, December 4, 2002

I made many telephone calls today to try and determine if we could get an oxygen concentrator at the timeshare in Villa Rica, Georgia. I began my effort by contacting Lincare, our present provider, then the time-share management in Georgia, plus a couple of other leads that were given to me. Getting oxygen probably could have been arranged but Muriel suggested it might be too taxing on her to make the trip, so we decided not to go. We ate dinner in the basement at church prior to the Advent service and Muriel directed the Chorale. Because of the COPD it was really difficult for her to get from the basement to the second floor, but she broke it into two segments as we practiced on the first floor and she had time to recover before climbing to the balcony. On the way home, I said, "You know, if I had my druthers I would prefer that you stay at home at this point and not tax your system to such a degree with all of the stair climbing."

"It's just for short periods of time that I am panting, and you see how quickly I recover."

"How did I know that's what you would say?"

"Because you know how much I like being the director of the Chorale, and how it is so fulfilling for me."

"I know sweetheart, I am just thinking of your well-being."

"I know, and I am grateful that you are."

Friday, December 6, 2002

Muriel was magnanimous in her desire to have me go skiing. So I called the Boston Mills Snowline and found out that they had a good base of man-made snow. Next stop for me, the Boston Mills ski area. I was back by 4:00 reinvigorated, and made dinner.

Wednesday, December 11, 2002

It was a very early morning for Muriel, as she was scheduled for a CT scan at 7:30. We left home before 7:00 to ensure that we wouldn't be late. I dropped her off at the entrance to the hospital and got her into a wheelchair, which I positioned well inside the lobby away from the doorway, and then I parked the car. I returned to the lobby and pushed her wheelchair to the check-in area and we reported our presence. Since the bone scan was scheduled at 8:00, we were able to convince the technician to leave the IV in place. The bone scan, as usual, required a second trip back to the hospital which we completed after lunch. In the evening, we ate dinner at church and then went to the Advent service. Because of public prayers on Sunday, many people asked Muriel how the tests went. However, since she just had the scans that day, we had no knowledge of what they will show.

Monday, December 16, 2002

This morning we had another appointment with Dr. Maggio. He had prescribed Levaquin to address Muriel's sinus infection and wanted her back for a check-up. I dropped Muriel off close to the entrance and quickly caught up with her so I could help her walk to the office. The nurse put us in an examination room and took Muriel's blood pressure (140/80). Dr. Maggio said, "Your blood pressure is down from the last visit. Did the Levaquin work?"

"Yes, my sinus infection has cleared up and all I have now is an occasional cough." She went on to say, "Dr. Koenig had ordered another bone scan and a CT scan which I had done last week." The doctor completed a physical examination, provided refill prescriptions of a number of medications, and suggested that she return in one to two months. I made an appointment for February 17, 2003 and we returned home. Pastor Larry came to visit Muriel in the afternoon and I felt she was uplifted by his presence, prayers, and concern for her well-being.

It has been said that persons who are dying have a sense that it is so, but may not necessarily have a grasp of how imminent it might be. During the last few weeks Muriel has updated the videos list and had gotten in touch with Dr. Reep, the chairperson of the English department at the University of Akron, to offer her the opportunity to select any videos that she judged the department would like to have. Muriel wanted to donate them to her former department while she was still alive. She also completed a list of books she was willing to donate to the Stow Public Library, and today I dropped off that list for them to check and let me know which books they would like. For dinner I made a big pot of bean soup using several ham bones as the base. It also had cut-up potatoes, carrots, celery, and onion. It will last us several days.

Wednesday, December 18, 2002

I called Dr. Koenig's office today to have a renewal prescription for Vicodin called into the CVS pharmacy, as Muriel's supply is nearly gone and she seems to be having more occurrences of pain. I did some wash and I even ironed, but Muriel was insistent that she would get around to ironing her own clothes later in the week. I made dinner for

Muriel and picked up the prescription on my way to church. Many at church asked after Muriel, and I indicated that her pain level seems to be on the rise. There were also several people who asked me how I am doing and whether I need any help. I assured them all that with Muriel's continued positive attitude I am doing just fine.

Thursday, December 19, 2002

Maybe bad news from a doctor should always be delivered face-to-face and directly to the patient. Then again, maybe that is not always possible. Dr. Koenig called me this morning and said, "Muriel's latest bone scan and CT scan indicate that additional tumors have been found on the ribs. Also, there is a lesion appearing on the liver." He went on to say, "At this time I am referring her to Visiting Nurse Service and placing her under hospice care. My concern for the present is to control Muriel's pain." I didn't ask specifically about the prognosis, but you could tell by the tone of his voice and the referral to hospice care that Muriel is not going to survive this latest cancerous assault on her body. I said, "I want to thank you and your staff for all of the care you have given Muriel."

After hanging up the telephone, I grasped the back of the chair beside me and let the gravity of what I had just heard sink in. Tears began to run down my cheeks and I had a brief flashback to the meditation area at church where Muriel first told me she had breast cancer. I thought about the peace she had prayed for and now I, too, asked God to send a special measure of His peace to both of us.

In a sense I am glad that I was the one to tell Muriel about the results of the tests. Considering the pain she is experiencing and the Vicodin she is taking to mask the pain, she knew that something was not right. I composed myself and waited for her to come downstairs for her morning cup of coffee, which I had prepared for her when I heard her first stirrings upstairs. She took up her usual position on the side of the table nearest the stove and I sat opposite her. "What is your level of pain this morning?"

"About a four."

"Dr. Koenig called with the results of your latest scans." I really didn't have to say much more because she knew from her body that new tumors had formed. We reached out with our hands across the table and I could not keep the tears from sliding down my cheeks once again. I eventually came around to her side of the table and knelt down and put my arms around her and said, "I love you with all of my heart." After we had a good cry together she said, "Tell me all about the telephone call."

"He said your latest bone scan and CT scan indicated that additional tumors have been found on the ribs and there is also a lesion appearing on the liver."

"I could tell by my pain that something new had cropped up."

"He is referring you to Visiting Nurse Service and is placing you under hospice care. He also said, 'My concern for Muriel is to control her pain.'"

"Did he give you a prognosis?"

"No, he didn't say anything, though I judge the referral to hospice implies an anticipated time frame."

I spent a portion of the afternoon making telephone calls. I talked with each of our children, giving them the latest information that was available. Each was saddened by the news, and both said to tell mom that they love her and they will be praying for her. I called Lois Jenkins, Muriel's Stephen Minister, who has been making monthly visits to support Muriel as she continues on her adventure. Robin Graham, the woman in her support group who has served as her driver to all of the support group activities, was next on my list. Robin was distraught at the news and assured me that she will come and visit Muriel within the next few days.

Saturday, December 21, 2002

I have often cooked over the nearly 44 years that we have been married, and even have two specialties that I am responsible for making: waffles and potato pancakes. In addition, since Muriel, I can say almost unequivocally, never cooks without the use of a recipe, I often did the cooking for us following a recipe she had selected. However, today for the very first time, following her pattern of arranging menus for the month, I made menus for the next two weeks. Having accomplished that, I can really appreciate what she does each month as she laid out all of the meals for each day.

Monday, December 23, 2002

I called Dr. Koenig's office this morning to let him know that the Vicodin is not doing a good job on Muriel's pain. He said, "I'll switch her to OxyContin. It's a drug used to treat moderate to severe pain. I'll start her with a 20 mg tablet that she'll take every 12 hours. In addition, I'll write a prescription for OxyIR 5 mg capsules that are to be taken every three to four hours for pain as needed."

"She also needs a renewal of the Kadian."

"I'll fax a renewal to the CVS pharmacy in Stow, but you'll have to come into the office to pick up the other two."

I concluded the IR stood for "Instant Relief" so I made a quick trip to 95 Arch Street to get the prescriptions. I then dropped them off at the same pharmacy where later, I would pick up all three.

Tuesday, December 24, 2002

Muriel and I went to the ten o'clock Christmas Eve candlelight service. I dropped her off at the front door and walked her inside where I helped her with her coat, and then got the wheelchair and seated her in it. I parked the car and returned to the vestibule, wheeled Muriel to the front of the church, and got her comfortable in the first pew. I was singing with the Chorale and would join her after we sang our anthem. As I sat in the balcony, many people went to the front of the church to talk with Muriel, as her worsening condition had been announced in public prayers on Sunday. After singing, I was coming downstairs with another member and I broke down in tears as the realization hit me that this may be the last Christmas we spend together. I gathered myself before I went into church to be with Muriel. There was an extra special closeness between us when we went to Communion. As we sat in the front pew, many people coming to Communion either leaned over and said something to her or just touched her on the shoulder as they went by. She always has had overwhelming support from the members of our congregation. We returned home for our usual Christmas Eve fare. However, we did cut back and we did not stay up as late.

Friday, December 27, 2002

Today we were visited by Patricia A. Pabst, licensed social worker, of Visiting Nurse Service (VNS) associated with hospice care. She was following up on Dr. Koenig's referral. We heard all about what VNS will be doing for Muriel, and there were a number of questions that needed to be answered and all of the forms that needed to be signed. She was accompanied by Gail Kubick, a registered nurse, who took care of the medical assessment so a proper care plan could be set up. I think the whole experience was rather tiring for Muriel, because when it got to the point of signing for having received the privacy notice she authorized me to sign it. There were several pages in the report filed by Gail Kubick. The table that follows represents her assessment and Muriel's concurrence of her own capability with the activities of daily living.

ACTIVITY OF DAILY LIVING	UP AS TOLERATED
Hygiene	Good
Bathing	Assisted 1 Person
Ambulation	Assisted 1 Person
Dress Upper	Assisted 1 Person
Dress Lower	Assisted 1 Person
Oral Hygiene	Independent
Grooming	Assisted
Shampoo	Assisted
Toileting	Assisted
Meal Preparation	Dependent
Eating	Independent
Medication Preparation	Dependent
Housekeeping	Dependent
Laundry	Dependent
Finance	Dependent
Shopping	Dependent
Telephone	Independent
Transport	Assisted 1 Person

Before the two representatives from hospice departed they shared that VNS would provide a large 4-inch foam pad for the bed and one for the chair where Muriel sits in the family room. Later on in the afternoon these pads were delivered to us. Each was put in its appropriate place and Muriel found the chair pad to be quite comfortable. The one on the bed also proved to be a comfort to her body. One can see from Muriel's discussion with the nurse that she has become increasingly dependent on me to do many of the things that were formally her purview.

Monday, December 30, 2002

At this stage I am still comfortable leaving Muriel by herself. So I prepared her pills for the day, and while she was still asleep I went to my morning breakfast Bible class and then played some social bridge with some seniors at the Quirk Center. When I returned home she was up and indicated to me that she was down to her last five Kadian and that maybe I should call hospice.

I made a call in the afternoon and informed Barbara Baird, RN, of the status of the Kadian. Barbara indicated that Susan Slagle, the visiting nurse assigned to Muriel, would come tomorrow and we should discuss it with her.

Tuesday, December 31, 2002

Today marked the first visit of Susan Slagle, the nurse from VNS. Susan endeared herself to us from the start. She is very personable and exhibits a take-charge demeanor. We are confident that if she, based on Muriel's assessment of pain, judges that her pain medication should be increased, that Dr. Koenig would ensure that it was so. Since control of pain was paramount for Muriel, she believes herself to be in good hands. Susan checked Muriel's blood pressure (130/72), pulse (88), and respirations (20), and listened to her heart. She then asked, "On a scale of zero to ten, what is your pain level?"

"It's a zero for my back, and about a five for my ribs."

"Tell me about your use of the OxyIR."

"I seem to be taking one every three hours."

"I am going to up your OxyContin to 40 mg every 12 hours, and I want you to carefully monitor the frequency of taking the OxyIR."

"I'll keep close track and I know Keith will keep watch also."

"I see you are on oxygen full-time. Is that helping your shortness of breath?"

"Initially I thought that being on oxygen full-time was going to be a problem, but I am glad that I am. However, any undue exertion just leaves me gasping for breath, but once I breathe the pure oxygen and rest, my breathing quickly returns to normal."

"You might want to consider upping the oxygen flow when you anticipate undue exertion."

Lastly, Susan made a call to Dr. Koenig's office and suggested the increase in OxyContin to 40 mg and also requested a renewal of the Kadian Muriel is taking. After a short wait she reported that he would fax the prescriptions to CVS and I could pick them up later in the afternoon. She had been with us for a little more than a half hour and I was confident that Muriel was in good hands.

After dinner tonight I bundled Muriel up and we went to the seven o'clock New Year's Eve service. We took Communion together and listened to many of our fellow churchgoers as they shared their concerns and cares for Muriel. We picked up the prescriptions on the way home from church and closed out the year with thanks to God for bringing Susan into our lives.

Thursday, January 2, 2003

We spent a quiet entry into the new year. However, today we renew the adventure. We had an appointment with Dr. Kretchmer, Muriel's pulmonologist. The Escort was filled from the liquid oxygen tank in the garage, Muriel was bundled up, and we drove into Akron. I parked in the deck and had Muriel stay in the car while I got a wheelchair to transport her to the office of Akron Pulmonary Associates. I signed her in, removed her coat, and wheeled her into the examination room. The nurse took her blood pressure (138/68), pulse (83), temperature (96°), and checked the oxygen level in her blood (92%). When Dr. Kretchmer came he asked, "How are you doing with the puffers?"

"I'm using the Atrovent, the Advair disks, and the albuterol, all of which seem to help me with my breathing." She added, "Lately I have been coughing, and it has produced a thick, yellow mucous. I think I am getting another sinus infection. Will you provide me with a prescription for Levaquin?"

"No problem. I'll give you that before you leave."

"Thank you." Muriel shifted in her wheelchair and continued, "I have really had difficulty breathing when over-exerting, like going upstairs. I am so quickly out of breath."

"I want you to increase the oxygen flow to five liters per hour when you over-exert, and then when the breathing is back to normal move it back to four liters per hour." He supplied us with a prescription for Levaquin, and we went from his office to Dr. Koenig's office, where I requested refills of the prescriptions for OxyContin and Kadian. Having accomplished that we returned home. I got Muriel comfortable in her recliner and set up a movie for her while I ran some other errands.

Later on in the afternoon I called Don and Ruth White and Bill and Nadine Gordon. I was amazed to find out that Don had died and no one had notified us. I expressed our condolences to Ruth and apologized for our failure to be at the funeral. We had been closely involved with each of these couples in our ministry in Marriage Encounter.

Bill and Nadine had been our workshop couple when we prepared our talks, and we had done several weekends together as presenting couples. We had also been on the same weekend team with Don and Ruth on several occasions. I wanted to let them know of Muriel's status on her adventure, and all of them expressed that they wished to come and visit her and will let me know the date they will be coming.

Friday, January 3, 2003

I put out the garbage, recycle bins, and lawn refuse on the curb after I exercised this morning. Because of the holiday we were delayed a day. I showered and then prepared my shopping list while we waited for Susan, the RN from VNS, to arrive for her 11:30 appointment.

I greeted Susan at the door and as I hung up her coat I said, "Since the increase in OxyContin, Muriel has been using only one capsule per day of the OxyIR."

"That's very good."

"I would really like to have a wheelchair for Muriel to minimize the amount of energy she expends to move about the house."

"Keith, your wish is my command." She got out her cell phone and requested immediately delivery of a wheelchair. It was at this point that she received a call requesting her presence elsewhere, so she left telling us that she would return in the afternoon. True to her word, at 1:40 she returned. She checked Muriel's blood pressure (118/68), pulse (80), and respirations (20). "I hear you're taking only one OxyIR pill a day."

"Yes, but sometimes I don't think that is enough."

"What are your pain levels now?"

"Right now I'm good with a zero for my back and a two for my ribs. However, sometimes between the OxyContin pills the pain level seems to be as high as seven or eight and more OxyIR would be good."

Susan immediately called Dr. Koenig's office and suggested that Muriel be permitted to take two to three capsules when breakthrough pain, the consistent stabbing pain in the eight to ten range, occurred in a 3-hour period. She said, "Dr. Koenig approved my suggestion and I would like you to maintain a record of the use of OxyIR. What about your shortness of breath?"

"Dr. Kretchmer, too, suggested that I up the flow of oxygen particularly when I am going upstairs." Some additional discussion ensued about bowel movements, eating habits, and her emotional status. She finished by listening to Muriel's breathing and her heart rhythms. She departed at 2:20.

I knew that Muriel would snooze, so I took the opportunity to do some errands. Since it was the beginning of the month, one of the errands was to do the grocery shopping. It was no fun without Muriel, and I am certain that I am not as efficient as she in arranging my list to coincide with the layout of the store. Needless to say, I did some serious backtracking. Maybe I'll get better at this. I also went to Sears and the Time Warner Cable office.

When I arrived at home, I put away the groceries and got out all of the ingredients to bake a pie. While I was making dinner the wheelchair was delivered. In the evening, Dave and Brenda Lietz, two of the members of the Chorale, called on Muriel to express their care and concern. Once they had departed it was time to get Muriel to bed and establish a routine, using the new wheelchair, in the process. I wheeled Muriel from the family room through the kitchen, dining, and living room area to the foot of the stairs. She then left the wheelchair, which I took to the top of the stairs, and then returned to the bottom to support her as she slowly inched up the stairs. When she reached the top she again seated herself in the wheelchair, and I took her to the bathroom where she brushed her teeth, went to the john, and then back into the wheelchair, and I wheeled her right to the bed. If she needed to get into her pajamas, I assisted. However, she often spends the day in pajamas and a robe, so it is only necessary to remove the robe.

Coming downstairs the following morning, we reversed the process, and there was not as much of a problem. I wheeled her to the top of the stairs and then carried the wheelchair down to the bottom. She sat on the top step and then bumped down the stairs, step by step. She took her time doing this, and was not winded when she reached the bottom. Then it was back into the wheelchair to the final destination, the family room and her recliner.

Tuesday, January 7, 2003

I did my usual exercises this morning and then exercised some more by shoveling out the driveway. About three inches of new snow fell overnight, and we had an appointment later in the day with Dr. Koenig. I ate breakfast, showered, and then got Muriel up. She showered and washed her hair. I had taken out the gooseneck shower spout and installed a flexible hose with a hand-held shower nozzle. We had also purchased a plastic footstool that was put in the shower so Muriel could sit while she was carrying out her ablutions. It worked really well, and I helped her into the shower, waited until she was done to help her out again, and then dried off her legs and back.

After lunch I got Muriel situated in the car and also placed the wheelchair in the trunk. It was much easier to use the one we had rather than having to go find one each time. We parked on the second deck and I wheeled Muriel directly to Dr. Koenig's office. The waiting room was partially filled. I hung up our coats and we soon were called to the examination room. She was weighed along the way (116 pounds) and then had her blood pressure taken (100/60) in the examination room. Dr. Koenig asked, "How are you doing on your pain medication?"

"Before I answer that, what is my prognosis?"

"I wish I could say otherwise, but you have, at best, three to six months."

With that information, I took a deep breath and let it out slowly. Muriel said, "I need to know because I have to make plans for my death. I'm not afraid of dying, but I don't want to leave any loose ends before I go. I also want to make sure that we minimize the pain I will endure."

"I assure you that we will do everything we can to make that happen. You are under hospice care and they will be checking with me on a regular basis to ensure that every measure we can take to relieve your pain is being implemented. There is no further need for the Aredia treatments and I want you to stop taking the Aromasin."

"I am experiencing pain levels that are often in the eight and nine range and maybe the OxyContin should be at a higher level."

"Let's raise the dosage to 60 mg every 12 hours. I'll give you a new prescription for that. You should also take four OxyIR capsules every two hours for breakthrough pain."

"I want to thank you for all that you have done for me, and I am still praying for a miracle."

"I would like to see you in a month or more."

I made an appointment for February 24, pretty positive that she will be able to keep it. When we got home I settled Muriel into her recliner and I went to do some errands. On my way I dropped off the prescription at CVS and then went to the Motor Vehicle Bureau to pick up a form to obtain a handicapped parking permit. Acme was next, to do a little grocery shopping, and later I picked up the prescription at CVS before returning home. Prior to making dinner, I began making telephone calls to all of the companies from which Muriel received catalogs, to cancel the mailings. The initial calls were made to the companies whose catalogs we had accumulated since Christmas. This routine will go on for many days as new catalogs arrive.

Wednesday, January 8, 2003

Midmorning I called Dr. Koenig's office to see if he was available to sign the form requesting a handicapped parking permit. He was in for the day, and after I got Muriel up and settled for the morning, I drove into Akron and went to his office to have him sign the form. From his office I drove directly to the Motor Vehicle Bureau to turn in the request and received the hanging placard. It will be much easier now getting Muriel from the car to wherever we may be going.

Friday, January 10, 2003

This morning I was doing lots of busy work around the house while waiting to get Muriel up. I have been sorting and cataloging bills and statements as I am getting together everything I need for my 2002 taxes. In addition, I am trying to update my financial statement that I prepare for Muriel each year as to our investments, our assets and liabilities, and who should be contacted for each area should anything happen to me. I have been doing this for the past ten years and Muriel really appreciated knowing all that information. It soon may become an exercise I do for my children.

Susan, from VNS, arrived after lunch. Meeting with her is like the experience we had with Dr. Doncals. She is so personable and so positive. She has a great sense of humor and a quiet demeanor as she goes about the task of examining Muriel. The basics indicated pulse (84), blood pressure (122/66), and respirations (24). She then asked, "What are your pain levels?"

"My back is a two and my ribs are a two. For the last several days, my appetite has really decreased. The food just doesn't taste good or the same as it used to."

"It's probably your cook." We all had a good laugh. "Experiment and find out what tastes good, and eat those foods."

"I saw Dr. Koenig on Tuesday and he took me off Aromasin and said there will be no more Aredia treatments. He also upped my OxyContin to 60 mg. When I asked for a prognosis, he told me I have approximately three to six months to live."

"That is just guess work."

"True, only God knows when I will die. I'm not afraid of dying, in fact I have made all of my final arrangements."

"Well, if you need me just call the office and they will page me."

Pastor Johnson came by later in the afternoon and visited with Muriel and then gave her Communion. For Muriel, having Communion is a source of strength as she continues on her adventure. I also participated, because sharing in the Lord's Supper with Muriel is very important for both her and me.

Saturday, January 11, 2003

It was cold outside, but Muriel wanted to go to the Akron Symphony Orchestra concert this evening. So I filled the Escort with oxygen from the tank in the garage, loaded the wheelchair in the car, and we departed. We left early enough that we parked under E. J. Thomas Hall and took the elevator to the lobby. I wheeled Muriel into the main entryway and we took another elevator to the mezzanine area. E. J. Thomas Hall accommodates wheelchair patrons in a section of Row C in the Grand Tier. Our season subscription seats are in the front row of the Grand Tier, but tonight we had the wheelchair in Row C and I found a seat nearby. Ya-Hui Wang was the conductor and selected *An American in Paris* by George Gershwin as the opening piece. It is a familiar piece and the orchestra played it well. The next two pieces were by the German-American composer Erich Wolfgang Korngold. The first was "Straussina," where the composer selected two obscure pieces by Leo Strauss and tied them together in a Straussian style. The second was a Violin Concerto in D Major, Op. 35, with Juliette Kang as the solo violinist. After intermission the orchestra played *Daphnis et Chloé* Suite No. 2 by Maurice Ravel. It was a wonderful concert, well played by the orchestra, and Muriel was happy she had braved the weather and attended.

Tuesday, January 14, 2003

Patti Peterson paid Muriel a visit yesterday. She is another Stephen Minister in our church. She spent about two hours with Muriel and it seemed to provide Muriel with an uplifting experience.

This morning, after I exercised, I did a tub of wash and ironed some shirts and jeans. At ten o'clock I assisted Muriel in getting downstairs where she moved onto her recliner. Shortly after she was up, the respiratory therapist from Lincare arrived to check how Muriel was doing. Muriel explained that Dr. Kretchmer had suggested that she bump up her oxygen flow to five liters per hour when she was subject to extra exertion. The therapist judged it would be better to maintain flow at that level all of the time. However, we were reluctant to do that unless directed to do so by Dr. Kretchmer. Thus, we will maintain the flow at the four liters per hour level.

Susan arrived a little after 2:00 and immediately began an assessment of Muriel's pain levels. Muriel said, "The pain level in the back is at a seven and the pain in the ribs is a two, and so far today I have taken two doses of five capsules each of OxyIR for the breakthrough pain."

"Let's see if we can raise the OxyContin level." Susan then called Dr. Koenig's office and spoke with Radhika Mullins, RN, to see if the OxyContin could be raised to 80 mg every 12 hours. While she waited for a call back from Radhika she measured Muriel's pulse (80), blood pressure (104/58), respirations (24), and oxygen saturation (96%). Next came the stethoscope and a check of the heart and lungs. Muriel got a thumbs-up on both. Just as she finished, Radhika called to say that the level of OxyContin would be raised to 80 mg, and he was also adding prednisone, 10 mg, to be taken twice daily. Those two prescriptions plus a renewal of the OxyIR would be faxed to the CVS pharmacy.

Susan asked, "How is your diarrhea these days?"

"I have been trying to wean myself off of the Kadian and I think my bowel is back working properly."

"Your stools are normal?"

"Yes, and I am having daily BMs even though I still am not eating regularly."

"That's good to hear. You take care. I will see you on Friday."

It amazes me that, for all of those months of diarrhea, now she is going off the Kadian and all is well. I waited an appropriate time and then went to CVS to pick up the new prescriptions. Much to my dismay the OxyContin was still at the 40 mg level, so between Muriel and me we decided she could take two of the pills and she would have 80 mg. We also knew that Susan would be back on Friday to see if the new medications are helping to cope with the pain.

Wednesday, January 15, 2003

Pastor Al came to visit Muriel today. He was an assistant pastor at our church several years ago but is now a chaplain at Stow Glen, a retirement community in Stow. He and his family are still members of our parish and we often see them in church. His wife Barbara used to sing in the Chorale, but as a result of a heart transplant she is now limited in her extracurricular activities. Pastor Al is a very personable individual and is well-liked by our membership. He made Muriel laugh as they chatted. She shared with him that she has included a part for him in her memorial service, and he said that he would be sad about losing her as a friend but he would be happy to participate.

Later in the day, Sue d'Amico, the pianist for the Chorale, stopped by to see Muriel. With Muriel's absence, Sue has become the de facto leader of the Chorale and Muriel is grateful for that. Sue brought Muriel a gift, which was a picture of an eagle in flight with its wings fully extended.

Muriel shared with Sue that she would like to have the Chorale sing at her memorial service. She spoke of the music she wanted to have, and they decided that they would get together later in the spring.

Friday, January 17, 2003

Susan arrived today at 2:00. The routine was almost a carbon copy of Tuesday. She carried her bag into the family room and asked Muriel, "What's your pain level?"

"It's a seven for the back and five for the ribs."

At that point I jumped in with, "When I went to pick up Muriel's prescription at CVS on Wednesday it was still at the 40 mg level, so we doubled the dosage to get to the 80 mg level that you had suggested and it still doesn't seem to be at a proper level."

"I don't want pain to run my life and I'd like better control. A level of two or three I could tolerate."

"Let's see what we can do about that."

Susan called Dr. Koenig's office and talked with Radhika Mullins and suggested that the dosage of OxyContin be increased to 120 mg. While waiting for the callback, she took Muriel's vital signs: pulse (84), respirations (24) and blood pressure (130/70). She checked her lungs and heart rhythms. "How's your appetite?"

"I think the prednisone has increased my appetite."

The callback from Dr. Koenig indicated that he would fax a new prescription for OxyContin 120 mg to be taken twice daily and that she should continue to use the OxyIR for breakthrough pain. Susan left at 3:20 and at 4:00 I went to the pharmacy to pick up the new prescription. Again, I was taken aback as the dosage was 80 mg. So when I got home I related this to Muriel, and we made the decision she would take one 40 mg tablet and one 80 mg tablet every 12 hours.

Saturday, January 18, 2003

Usually after Muriel is up and has had her first cup of coffee, she sets up her pills for the rest of the day and the following morning. I judged that she is really taxed to keep them in order, and I offered to take over the daily pill preparation. I had offered before, but she seemed to be reluctant to let me do it. However this morning she readily agreed to let me add that task to my daily regimen.

Wednesday, January 22, 2003

We had a new visitor today: Shirley Hayes, an RN from hospice, who is a pain specialist. Shirley came because there has been difficulty in getting the pain medications set to Muriel's satisfaction. She was with us for nearly two hours, and quizzed Muriel extensively on the levels of pain in her back and ribs and how it felt. Did it move? Was it constant? She seemed to get a good reading from Muriel and she recommended to Dr. Koenig that she start taking Neurontin, a prescription medicine used to treat nerve pain, which he approved at a level of 100 mg. She took Muriel's vital signs: pulse (88), respirations (20), and blood pressure (146/86). She also checked her heart and lungs.

After lunch Marjorie Riehl and Marie House, two ladies from our church, came to visit with Muriel. Marjorie had breast cancer some time ago, but in her case it had not metastasized. While they chatted I went to CVS to pick up the new prescription and added it to the collection of medications Muriel was taking. My pick-up also included a renewal of the OxyIR.

Friday, January 24, 2003

Muriel has said that the use of the Neurontin has really helped and she is feeling much better. In fact, she insisted that I get out and go skiing. I honored her request and went to Boston Mills and skied from the opening until just after 1:00. Susan was coming in the afternoon and I wanted to be there to be of any help and to listen to Muriel express her joy at what the Neurontin had done.

Susan arrived at 2:45 and began with the usual check of the vital signs: pulse (72), blood pressure (138/78), and respirations (20). Next she checked her heart and lungs. "So how is your pain?" Susan asked. Muriel was happy to provide the levels of pain, "For the back it is zero and for the ribs it is one. I think with the Neurontin I now have control over my pain and we can maintain it at a tolerant level."

After Susan had departed, Betty Dodd came to visit Muriel. She too has experienced breast cancer, and is now considered a survivor as she has made it past the five-year mark. Betty is one of the faithful members of the church who practices a card ministry. Her cards always arrive at just the right time to give Muriel an extra boost. After dinner, Chuck and Nancy Segner came to visit with Muriel and me. Chuck and Nancy were our prayer couple on our first Marriage Encounter weekend, which gives them a specialness in our lives. By the time they departed Muriel was bushed, and I got her upstairs and into bed.

Tuesday, January 28, 2003

We watched the Super Bowl on Sunday. I made a seven-layer Mexican dip that we ate with Doritos. It was probably not good for either of us, but we thoroughly enjoyed it. Today Muriel stepped out on her own with the help of Robin Graham. She and several of the members of the cancer support group had lunch together. I suggested to Robin that she take the wheelchair with her, as it would be easier for Muriel to get around, which she did. When she returned, about three hours later, she was pumped up. I think she was feeling the same way as I do when I return from skiing. I said a prayer of thanks that she was able to have this time with her friends.

I did errands while Muriel was out. One place I visited was the Country Inn in Cuyahoga Falls. It may be premature, but the three to six month prognosis dictates that each of our children and their families journey to Ohio and bid a loving farewell to their mother and grandmother, so I was checking on costs and availability of accommodations.

Thursday, January 30, 2003

Today marks the 44th anniversary of our life together as a married couple. Since the Neurontin has helped with Muriel's pain and the prednisone has helped with her appetite, I decided that we would have our usual anniversary dinner. After she had gotten up, we shared the common anniversary card and a cup of coffee, and then I went to Acme to pick up all the ingredients for the dinner. In the afternoon I went and played bridge with the group at church and Muriel welcomed Sue d'Amico and Rita Cargill, the office secretary at church, for a visitation. After bridge I made our anniversary dinner: Duckling Rosé, wild rice, and asparagus. We had tapioca pudding with Cool Whip for dessert. We ate at the dining room table and we lingered over the meal, finished off the bottle of wine, and reflected on the 44 years we had shared.

When Muriel experienced the first metastasis she wanted us to get to our 50th anniversary, and right now it looks like we are not going to reach that goal. We talked about the birth of our children and how she had made it easy on me way back then, as I did not have to wait endless hours for them to be born. Mark was born in Potsdam, New York on December 22, 1959. I was a junior in college at the time and was working for the university cleaning dorm rooms over the Christmas break. I had come home for lunch and Muriel told me her water had broken and we should go to the hospital. Her bag was packed, but I decided to check the Christmas cards from that day's mail as she stood there waiting. Dumb! We finally were on our way, and during the drive she had a contraction that nearly doubled her up. So we hustled to the hospital and I got her admitted to the delivery area. I told her I was going back home to shower and change my clothes and I would be back before she delivered. Well, as you can guess, Mark had arrived before I returned. So no pacing and no anxiety for me.

On February 27, 1962, the day that Kay was born, I had already left the apartment and caught the bus in Palisades Park, New Jersey on my way to the Port Authority in NYC, and then took the subway to my job with the New York Telephone Company. At 10:00 I received a call from my mother-in-law telling me that Grandpa had just left with Muriel to drive her to Englewood Hospital, as our second child was on the way. I immediately left work and reversed my journey back to our apartment, where I picked up my car and drove to the hospital. However, Kay had already been born. They had even delayed the birth so some student nurses could be available to watch, and I still didn't make it in time. I had always wanted to have four children, but after two breech births, Muriel said that I would have to have the next two.

We shed some tears and later talked about our grandchildren. It was not a regret, but Muriel expressed a concern that with our families living in the Dallas area and us in Ohio, we just didn't get to spend much time with them. It is really tough to have your grandchildren get to know you and build a relationship when you spend only about 20 days together out of the year and they come in three, four, and five-day blocks. When we finished, I helped Muriel upstairs and got her into her bed. It is probably going to be the first of many nights I have the opportunity to grieve while she is still alive. We are also experiencing many "lasts," and today appears likely to be the last anniversary we will celebrate together.

Friday, January 31, 2003

Patricia Pabst, a social worker associated with hospice, made a visit. Her write-up of her visit follows:

I had received a call late last week from husband regarding some questions over the couple's long-term care insurance. So today spent time looking at his policy. Pt has no waiting period and does have a reimbursement for daily care in the home. However, it is not clear who the insurance will accept to provide this care. As pt doing fairly well at present, husband chose to table further investigation of this care until the time it is needed. Pt had gotten out to her support group and a luncheon on Tuesday. The couple have been very pleased with present pain management. In fact, she wants husband to plan a ski trip and she will go along just to read. Husband told worker that wife never did enjoy skiing or bridge which are two of his hobbies; however, they did both enjoy golf and visited many of the well-known golf resorts in their travels.

Susan also visited and began with the vital signs: pulse (84), blood pressure (130/74), and respirations (24). Next came the pain measurements: back (zero) and ribs (zero). She also checked her heart and lungs. "I guess I can stop coming if we have your pain under control."

"No, no, I want to have someone who is keeping track of me."

"I'm just kidding you."

"I am pleased at what all of the pain medications have done. I told Keith to plan a week away so he could go skiing. I'll just read and relax."

"That would be a great idea."

"Last night we celebrated our 44th wedding anniversary. Keith prepared our traditional dinner and we reminisced about life together. We had a good cry when we discussed that it could very well be our last. However, I always pray that God will provide a miracle and we will make it to our 50th."

"It is good that you talk about your prognosis, but I'm with you, praying can be rewarding."

"I also met with my support group last Tuesday and had a wonderful time. I told them I would probably be the next to die, but that I am living every day to the fullest."

"Good for you." Susan departed shortly thereafter and seemed really excited for Muriel's euphoria. Just after dinner Muriel had two visitors, Bea Amos and Mary Currier. Way back, Muriel and I used to bowl in a couples league with Bea and her husband Dallas as our teammates. Bea was our anchorperson, as she is a very good bowler. Mary is a long-standing friend and has worked with Muriel on several committees at church. They were here for about an hour and a half. I am grateful for all the people who come to visit, but I judge I need to monitor their length of stay so Muriel is not exhausted at the end of the day. However, with all of the medication she is taking, she has no difficulty sleeping.

Tuesday, February 4, 2003

So far this month, Muriel's pain has been held in check with 120 mg of OxyContin taken twice daily and the 200 mg of Neurontin taken every eight hours. She has used little or no OxyIR, as there has been very little breakthrough pain. She is spending her time writing notes of thanks and encouragement to persons from whom she has received cards and for the persons who have visited her. I baked a cherry pie with a lattice-top crust today, and sent a confirmation of the reservation for the visit of Mark and his family in March. Susan, our ever-faithful hospice nurse, also was scheduled to see Muriel. She arrived at 3:30 and was with us for slightly less than an hour. She did her usual thing, pulse (80), blood pressure (128/70), and respirations (20). Pain scores were both zero for the back and ribs. Susan checked her lungs and heart as well. She then offered Muriel a home health assistant who would help her bathe, wash her hair, and take care of any other ablutions. Muriel declined the offer, judging that between the two of us everything is being taken care of.

Wednesday, February 5, 2003

Art Tischler, a friend and elder from church, stopped in yesterday to give us Communion, which is always an uplifting experience for both of us. Bill and Nadine Gordon together with Ruth White, dear friends from our ministry together in Marriage Encounter, visited us today. Nadine arrived in a wheelchair, and since I had wheeled Muriel to the front door while Nadine rolled down the ramp and Bill brought her onto the porch, the first few minutes were taken up with a wheelchair comparison. It just got the visit off to a beautiful beginning and Muriel immensely enjoyed the whole time they shared with her. Each visit that someone makes to see her is very poignant for her. *Is it the last time I will see this person?* appears to be the question that lingers in the air.

Friday, February 7, 2003

If she could have, I think Muriel would have booted me out of the house and onto the ski slope this morning. As she has been throughout this adventure, she just wants me to lead a normal life. "Play bridge," she says. "Go skiing." I honor her requests and get reinvigorated through these activities, which allows me the opportunity to better care for her. So this morning I was in the lift line when the slopes opened, and skied until noontime.

Susan was in at 1:50. Muriel's vital signs were recorded: pulse (80), blood pressure (138/80), and respirations (20). "What are your pain levels today?"

"It's zero for the back and one for the ribs." After checking Muriel's heart and lungs, Susan said, "Everything sounds good. Do you have any concerns today?"

"Taking the prednisone has certainly increased my appetite, but the result is an increase in my weight also, and the problem is that it looks like all of the weight has gone to my face. Using the steroid has also been helpful to my breathing, but I would like to get off of it."

"One of the side effects of prednisone is what is known as 'pie face.' We could begin to lower the dosage. Let's drop it to 10 mg and see what happens."

"We are going to the ballet tonight, so I took some Milk of Magnesia as I usually have a bowel movement in the evening."

"That's good, that follows the bowel regimen we set up when you stopped taking the Kadian. Enjoy the ballet."

I filled the Escort and we went to the ballet in the evening. It was held at E. J. Thomas Hall, so I parked Muriel's wheelchair in the same place that we had for the symphony orchestra concert, Row C in the Grand Tier. I think Muriel is very pleased with the portable oxygen and the knowledge that she can go out of the house with no consequences.

Tuesday, February 11, 2003

Susan arrived at 2:50 for Muriel's check-up. Each time she visits it is like having a member of your family come in. In her subtle way she asks questions about our lives and relationship and therefore gains a greater understanding of us, which probably helps her to better deal with us. Muriel's vitals were taken: pulse (84), blood pressure (134/74), and respirations (20). She listened to Muriel's heart and lungs and then checked the current pain levels for the back and ribs, both of them at a one. Muriel judged that the reduction to 10 mg of prednisone was good, as her appetite was still up and she still had a good energy level.

Wednesday, February 12, 2003

I had an appointment with my urologist this morning and then ran several errands on my way home. I made muffins, a very healthy recipe I had gotten from our daughter. They included oat bran, flaxseed, two apples, four carrots shredded, raisins, mixed nuts, and other spices. The recipe made two dozen muffins. A muffin and a small dessert cup of the fruit mix I make has become a staple for lunch for both Muriel and me. The fruit mix includes peaches, pears, pineapples, kiwis, red grapes, and oranges, and on the day that we have it I generally cut up a banana as well. After lunch Muriel said, "I want you to go skiing."

"I should be here to take care of you."

"I'm not dying yet, and before you go, please bring up the ironing board and iron from the basement, plus my blouses so I can iron them."

"Why don't you let me do your blouses?"

"There'll come a time when I will be happy to have you do them, but right now I want you to go skiing. Trust me that I wouldn't send you off if I wasn't confident that everything will be all right."

So I did as she requested, gave her a hug and a kiss, and went skiing. In the evening I went to Chorale practice. It just didn't seem right without Muriel up front directing.

Friday, February 14, 2003

Today is Valentine's Day and I left a card on Muriel's side of the table, awaiting her arrival for her morning cup of coffee. Susan came at 1:40 and was with us for an hour. All of the routine items were taken care of: pulse (84), blood pressure (138/84), and respirations (24). Pain levels were recorded: back (one) and ribs (zero). She checked her heart and lungs and concluded that everything was in working order.

Monday, February 17, 2003

I went to Bible class this morning and when I returned I shoveled the driveway and sidewalks. After lunch I brought Muriel to see Dr. Maggio for a routine visit. Muriel gave him all of the details regarding her hospice care and the extent of her medications. She had her blood pressure taken (136/74) and he listened to her heart and lungs. They talked about her use of the inhalers and whether they were working, which got a positive response from Muriel. Her basic problem is with exertion, which exacerbates the problem of breathing, so he concluded that she should cool it. Each day seems to be the end of something, and it is noted that today could be Muriel's last visit to her primary care physician.

Tuesday, February 18, 2003

This was a chance encounter day. I visited Falls Music in Cuyahoga Falls to check on some music that Muriel wanted to have played during her memorial service. Yes, it is February and Muriel has planned her whole memorial service—what music would be played, what hymns would be sung, the text for the sermon by Pastor Johnson and other Bible verses to be read by the liturgist. She also designated the participants in the service—Pastor Larry as liturgist and eulogist, Pastor Al as the Communion officiant, and Dave Lietz to sing the Deacon's Prayer. She wanted the Chorale to sing two numbers and she had selected four poems to be read. The readers would include two members of her support group, Robin Graham and Sue Wells, plus Lois Jenkins, her Stephen Minister, and our son Mark.

Muriel had asked me to find sheet music for "The Twelfth of Never," "Through the Years," and the Henry Mancini piece "Softly as I Leave You," which were to be played as pre-service music. I was standing in line and it was obvious by the conversation of the woman in front of me that she was a piano teacher. So I asked her how she liked teaching adults. She gave me a very enthusiastic response and introduced herself as Georgia Pawlowski, and gave me her business card. So I told her of the situation I am in with Muriel, and that when she passes away I will get in touch with her to see about taking lessons. I had always wanted to learn to play the piano. When I retired I found a computer program that consisted of a set of five CDs that held ten lessons each and I began practicing. I was very diligent, practicing one hour per day. After Muriel retired she would often watch and listen to me and made the observation that I was only playing chords with my left hand and not reading the specific notes. Since she played the piano she agreed to teach me. We got some adult piano books from the teacher who had taught our daughter and we began. We were somewhat successful, but then Muriel got cancer and the piano lessons were put on hold.

Susan visited Muriel in the afternoon. It was pretty routine, with pain levels estimated to be one and zero with respect to her back and ribs. Muriel did indicate she was taking two OxyIR capsules toward the end of the 12-hour cycle of the OxyContin. Muriel's vitals were taken: pulse (76), blood pressure (140/82), and respirations (28). Her lungs were clear and her heart was maintaining a normal rate and rhythm. Susan once again offered a home health attendant to help Muriel wash her hair and bathe. Muriel declined.

Friday, February 21, 2003

I used the morning to make a new batch of muffins and also went to Acme to do some grocery shopping. I have not been as efficient as Muriel with regard to shopping. Susan came right after lunch with her visit playing out nearly identically to her visit on Tuesday. The pain levels were very similar and the vital signs varied just slightly: pulse (84), blood pressure (124/74), and respirations (24).

In the afternoon I administered Communion for Muriel. Having been an elder in years past, I have been "officially" authorized to give Communion to Muriel. Later in the afternoon Ruth Towsey came to visit Muriel. Ruth is a dear friend who played in the Bell Choir at church at the same time that Muriel and I were members. She always sits in the pew in church just in front of the one that Muriel and I share. The two of them had a nice couple of hours.

Saturday, February 22, 2003

We spent a quiet day today, ate dinner at home, and then went to the Akron Symphony Orchestra concert. The music director selected two pieces by Beethoven. The program opened with Piano Concerto No. 3 in C Minor, Op. 37. Roberto Plano was the solo pianist, who exhibited a flawless technique. Because of the position of our regular seats, more readily able to observe the soloist, Muriel chose to sit in those seats, so we used the wheelchair to get to the entrance of the auditorium and then left it on the landing. The second half of the program was Symphony No. 3 in E-flat Major, Op. 55, commonly known as *Eroica*. It was an interesting selection because it is deemed that the writing of *Eroica* coincided with Beethoven's writing of his last will and testament. Beethoven is one of Muriel's favorite composers, so she enjoyed the concert immensely. We waited until the crowd had diminished and then worked our way back to the car. It was a good day and evening.

Monday, February 24, 2003

I went to Bible class and then played bridge with a group at the Quirk Center in Cuyahoga Falls. When I returned home I shoveled the driveway and sidewalk. After lunch, Muriel had an appointment with Dr. Koenig. Afternoon appointments are always good because there is little waiting time. I loaded the wheelchair in the car, as it would be easier to transport Muriel from the parking deck to the doctor's office. She got out of the chair to be weighed and registered as 134½ pounds, a significant increase from her last visit that could probably be allayed to the prednisone she is taking. Then it was back into the chair and into the examination room for her blood pressure (140/80). Upon entry Dr. Koenig asked, "How are you doing with pain control?"

"At the moment I have no complaints with regard to the dosage of the medications controlling my pain, but what upsets me is the weight I have gained."

"I would like you to taper off the prednisone. Let's reduce it to 2.5 mg every day for a week, and if you do well you can do 2.5 mg every other day for another week, and then stop completely." After his physical examination of Muriel, he suggested that she return in six months.

Tuesday, February 25, 2003

Today was "cleaner day," so we put our house in order, had lunch, and then we departed to go to the movies. We went to the Plaza 8 at Chapel Hill and after the movie we went to Applebee's for dinner. We stretched the limit of the Escort today, but we still got in under the wire. Muriel was maneuvering pretty well and judged she could do even better if she didn't have all of the weight she was carrying. The prednisone certainly keeps her appetite up. After dinner we returned home, refilled the Escort, and went to Chorale practice. We arrived early enough that she took her time getting up the stairs. Everyone was surprised to see her there. She didn't direct but just observed.

< 15 >
THE "ADVENTURE" IS WINDING DOWN

Saturday, March 1, 2003

After Muriel got up this morning, I stripped the beds and washed the sheets. When the sheets were dry I reversed the process, so that if Muriel wanted to return to bed, it was ready for her. Shirley Hayes, the pain specialist from VNS, came today at noontime. She was here mainly to make a new assessment of Muriel's pain and gather as much information as possible. Initially she took Muriel's vital signs: pulse (80), blood pressure (148/76), and respirations (28). She then said, "Tell me about your pain. I want you to give me a location, then on a scale of one to ten, the present level and the level at its worst."

"I'll start with my left rib area. Currently it's a zero with a worst level of three. The pain in that area is well-controlled. In my upper back, the numbers are zero and eight. These pains are mainly stabbing and shooting, occurring primarily in the morning, and can be dissipated with five OxyIR tablets. In my lower back the numbers are zero and six. It is a general aching pain that is sometimes aggravated by standing and bending forward to put on make-up."

"That's a pretty thorough analysis. Thank you for the information. Are you experiencing any shortness of breath?"

"I have shortness of breath whenever I have undue exertion, and it occurs mainly when I climb a flight of stairs. When I am moving in the house and when I'm outside the house I use the wheelchair."

"Let's go in another direction. Your skin looks good."

"I have been taking a shower at least once a week, and after I dry off Keith helps me put moisturizer all over my body."

"I read Susan's report that you had reduced the dosage of prednisone because of blurred vision."

"The blurred vision was primarily on distance, but it was annoying and the reduction to 2.5 mg has helped to clear that up."

"Is there anything else I should know?"

"Sometimes my incisions itch and even grab, but it's not really a problem because it usually stops. It often feels like the interior of my right arm is numb. Is there a prescription to help me lose 15 pounds? But maybe the extra weight helps me to sleep better."

"We all want to lose 15 pounds, Muriel, and perhaps you are sleeping better as a result. Is there anything else, any concerns outside your physical well-being?"

"I do have a concern for my sister in Texas. She had a heart valve replaced and that caused her scleroderma to return, which has led to the need for kidney dialysis. The best I can do is keep in touch by telephone. But the question really is, which one of us will be the first to die?"

"I think you have to let God be your guide on this."

"I know, I asked God to give me peace at the outset of this adventure and that peace continues to sustain me. In addition, I attend a support group once a month and there are four of us from the group that also meet for lunch on a regular basis. Members of my congregation have given me great support, and Keith has been phenomenal in the way he cares for me, so God is definitely in charge."

"That's great to hear. You really are blessed to have so much support. Thank you, Muriel, for inviting me into your home and giving me so much information. It will be really helpful in managing your pain." As she prepared to leave she added, "I enjoyed my first visit with you and this one has been great also."

Shirley was very thorough and I think Muriel was pretty exhausted by the time she left. After dinner this evening, Jill Williams, a member of our church, dropped in to visit with Muriel and offer encouragement.

Monday, March 3, 2003

Today, Mary McDaniel, an RN from VNS, came to see Muriel since Susan is on vacation. She initially checked Muriel's vital signs: pulse (96), blood pressure (124/72) and temperature (98.4°). After she was done,

I said, "After the visit from Shirley Hayes last Saturday, the midnight dosage of Neurontin was increased to three capsules. It does appear to be helpful, because Muriel does not have the breakthrough pain first thing in the morning that she had been experiencing in the past. However, the increased dosage appears to produce a side effect in that Muriel seemed 'out of it.' She has been sluggish and has difficulty getting her thoughts together. Her speech is slurred and she is sleeping more, even at meal times. Please have Shirley Hayes call me. We have to get this straightened out."

"Certainly. I'll have her call you."

"Thank you."

At dinnertime this evening I handed Muriel a cup of coffee, and rather than grasp it with both hands she tried to hold it with the cup handle alone. Well, the cup slipped and we had coffee all over Muriel. Fortunately it was not scalding hot and did little damage, but it was necessary to strip her and get clean, fresh pajamas and a robe for her. Perhaps the little incident startled her into reality, as she seemed to be her usual self. "So what happened there?" I asked.

"I guess I didn't have a firm grip on the cup."

"I think it was more than that. I think the increase in the Neurontin has made you a little spacey."

"I have felt a little disoriented."

"Okay, here's what I suggest we do. It's back to just two Neurontin at midnight, and if you have breakthrough pain in the morning at the end of your cycle, I will give you OxyIR according to the scale we devised."

"That's a good idea. We'll try it. Thank you sweetie. I thank God daily that you are here to care for me."

Kay and Kaitlyn planned on arriving later in the week, so I called Dr. Koenig's office to determine if it was okay for them to come since Kaitlyn has mononucleosis. Dr. Koenig gave the okay as long as there was not any close personal contact or the sharing of any eating utensils. So I called Kay and left a message on her answering machine that her trip is a go. As we had agreed earlier, at midnight Muriel returned to taking two 100 mg Neurontin capsules.

Thursday, March 6, 2003

Today we had another new RN from VNS named Kathryn Stack, who was covering for Susan. She took Muriel's vital statistics: pulse (80), blood pressure (126/64) and respirations (16). "What can you tell me about your pain?"

"The pain level for both my back and ribs are a zero. However, the pain in my back is at its worst in the morning when I first get up, and today it was at a ten. I immediately took five OxyIR capsules to mask the pain."

She then explained all about the change in the Neurontin and the setting up of a sliding scale for taking the OxyIR. She listened to Muriel's heart and lungs and then she was on her way.

Shortly after Kathryn departed, Kay and Kaitlyn arrived to spend some time with Oma and to officially say goodbye. Because both of our children work, Muriel and I had thought it best if each of them, together with the members of their family, visit before Muriel is incapacitated and unable to recognize them, or appreciate their presence. So Kay was the first to come. Larry and Kenton chose to remain at home. I made one of Kay's favorites for dinner, a hot green bean and sliced potato dish with a crumbled French-fried onion topping. I also heated up a turkey ham and we ate in the dining room and just enjoyed each other's company. At the end of the night, Kay and Kaitlyn retired to the third bedroom.

Saturday, March 8, 2003

After Muriel had taken her morning pills and had a cup of coffee, she had me bring down all of her jewelry. It was giveaway time. She couldn't just give it all to Kay and Kaitlyn, as she has a daughter-in-law and two other granddaughters to think of as well, but both her daughter and her first granddaughter fared very well. Kay was the recipient of Muriel's pearls, a diamond dinner ring, and several tennis bracelets, each with different stones. She also received the charm bracelet, a very special piece that represents Muriel's life in the 32 charms which are attached to it. Kaitlyn also got a diamond ring, a pass-down from Muriel's mom, plus other assorted rings and trinkets on chains.

Later in the evening Kay and I drove to the Nationwide Arena in Columbus where Kay's hometown team, the Dallas Stars, were playing the Columbus Blue Jackets in an NHL hockey game. It was a pleasant ride back to Munroe Falls, as the Stars won the game. When we arrived we found Muriel was still up and Kaitlyn was keeping her company, although they both looked like they had been snoozing.

Monday, March 10, 2003

I went to my usual Bible class breakfast this morning and then played some bridge. Shortly after I got home, Susan arrived. We chatted briefly and I introduced her to Kay and Kaitlyn, and then she went straight to work. She first took Muriel's vital signs: pulse (80), blood pressure (102/68), and respirations (20). She next listened to her lungs and heart, then asked, "What are your levels of pain?"

"Right now it's a zero in my back and a zero in my ribs."

I said, "The pain seems to be controlled, but we are concerned that she seems to be weaker, and she is less steady when she walks."

"Keith has to help me more as I move from place to place."

I continued, "When we talk she has difficulty finding the right words she wants to say and has trouble finishing sentences."

"All of these differences from what is normal for you are indications of the progression of the disease," Susan said.

"What about the difficulty breathing and the double vision?" I asked.

"The breathing problem is probably associated with her COPD, and the double vision may be from the medications," Susan responded.

"All I know is I have difficulty gathering my thoughts and finishing sentences. This is all new to me, as I'm usually a very articulate person. I decided to increase my dosage of prednisone back to the 10 mg level."

"You sound pretty good right now. Increasing the prednisone will probably return some of the strength you may have lost," Susan said.

I asked, "Did you get any feedback from your replacements?"

"There wasn't much in the notes."

"Well I made a decision, with Muriel's agreement, to reduce the three Neurontin pills taken at night to just two. She was really spacey and had difficulty holding a cup unless it was with both hands."

Muriel added, "I seemed to act more normally although there was an increase in the pain in the morning at the end of the cycle."

I said, "But we just countered that with the OxyIR according to our sliding scale."

Susan smiled and then added, "Well, you guys have apparently ironed it all out by yourselves." Before she departed she indicated that she would have Shirley Hayes fax a note to Dr. Koenig with an update of Muriel's condition.

Thursday, March 13, 2003

Kay and Kaitlyn made a tearful departure for Texas this morning with long hugs and declarations of love for mother and grandmother. Muriel has seemed less lethargic the last couple of days. The three of them had taken the opportunity to share and reminisce, with the emphasis on making this time together, likely their last, as pleasant and uplifting as possible.

After they had departed I filled the Escort with oxygen, packed Muriel and her wheelchair in the car, and drove to City Hospital. We had an appointment at 10:00 with Dr. Doncals. Since we had the wheelchair, I took Muriel across the bridge on the second floor and then took the elevator to the main floor and the radiation therapy department. We had just gotten our coats off when we were taken to an examination room. Dr. Doncals entered shortly and was her usual ebullient self. Between Muriel and me, we provided an update on Muriel's current condition. I'm sure that Dr. Doncals knows that Muriel's life is waning. However, she performed a thorough examination and when she was done we departed.

Friday, March 14, 2003

We began to make preparations for the Sunday arrival of Mark and his family. Although they are to stay at the Country Inn in Cuyahoga Falls, they will be sharing meals with us. Ever since Muriel returned to the 10 mg level for the prednisone, she has been back to her usual self. She showered this morning while I stood by to assist in the transfer of the cannula, and getting her in and out of the shower. She also weighed herself and the scale read 125 pounds, which is down, but much higher than she would have liked. As a result of getting all cleaned up and the change in medication, she was pretty chipper when Susan arrived at 1:30. Her vital signs were recorded: pulse (76), blood pressure (122/80), and respirations (24). Susan checked her lungs and heart and discussed pain levels, which were currently at an acceptable level of two for both her back and her ribs. Susan summed up her visit by saying, "You certainly are more alert and not having any trouble finishing your sentences today. I guess the increase in the prednisone is a good thing."

"I certainly feel I am more coherent. Thank you for your help."

"My pleasure."

Saturday, March 15, 2003

After Muriel woke up I stripped the beds and washed the sheets. When they were dry I remade the beds. Muriel is doing really well with pain control, but the COPD is causing her some difficulty, particularly when she expends any kind of energy. I helped her shower and dress (it is tough pulling up those pantyhose) and after dinner we went to E. J. Thomas Hall and were entertained by PDQ Bach. The highlight was his original composition, *The 'Battered' Bride*. Have oxygen and wheelchair, will travel. You have to be a fan of Richard Boone as Paladin to appreciate the comment.

Muriel seemed pumped up when we got home, but she was also nearing the end of a pain cycle and was beginning to feel stabbing pains in her back. She took four OxyIR capsules and within minutes the pain had subsided to level one. I had a cup of coffee and we sat in the family room and talked. She is very concerned about her sister and has called her several times in the past couple of weeks. We are not going to make a trip to Texas to see Judith, and because of dialysis Judith is not going to make the trip to Munroe Falls to see Muriel. The only lifeline for each of them is the telephone. She took her midnight pills, and I assisted her in climbing the stairs and put her to bed.

Sunday, March 16, 2003

We went to church this morning and celebrated Holy Communion together. Many members of the congregation came to have a word with Muriel. Listening to all of the well wishes and evidences of prayers for Muriel was a very uplifting time for her as well as for me. I still am getting asked how I am doing and I always reply the same. "With Muriel's positive attitude, the adventure moves forward, and I am just trying to keep up."

Mark and his family arrived late afternoon after they had checked into the Country Inn. In anticipation of their arrival I had made a big pot of chili and had gotten a loaf of sourdough bread. I think the latter was for me, as everybody else ate crackers. Sourdough bread is also good with peanut butter. Maybe I did get the bread for me.

After I cleaned up from dinner we had tiramisu cake with coffee. We got reacquainted with Emma Catherine, now 4½, and spent a quiet evening talking about their trip from Texas and how the girls are doing in school. They were tired from the trip and left for the motel at around nine o'clock.

Monday, March 17, 2003

It is St. Patrick's Day and I gave Muriel a card that I had gotten on an earlier errand. She is definitely an Anglophile, but that does not necessarily mean she is Irish-bent as well. However, she enjoyed the card. Mark and Cathy, with children, arrived just before lunchtime, so I made everybody grilled cheese sandwiches, some with lunch meat and some plain. After lunch, Muriel took all of the ladies in tow and proceeded to give away the rest of her jewelry. Later in the day I called Don Kraus, my insurance agent, to cancel the policy I had on the jewelry Muriel had passed down. Strike while the iron is hot. We sat around the rest of the afternoon and talked. Muriel brought everybody up to date of where she is on her adventure. I put together Chicken Divan for dinner. Everybody liked the chicken and rice, but not everyone ate the broccoli. Mark indicated that tomorrow he would be showing his family the area and all of his old haunts. I suggested they come by at 4:00 so they could meet Susan, and they departed a little before 9:00.

Tuesday, March 18, 2003

I had a busy morning. It began with a breakfast with Pastor Al. We have been meeting periodically to bolster each other as caregivers to our respective wives. I had served as his Stephen Minister when his wife Barbara initially had her heart transplant, and we have drawn close to each other to a point where we can shed tears and give each other a hug when we meet and when we part. It is always an uplifting time for me. When I returned home I made a butterscotch walnut pie, one of Mark's favorites. We also were out of muffins, so I prepared a new batch for lunches for Muriel and me. At 1:15 we had an appointment with Dr. Kretchmer.

I brought along Muriel's wheelchair so I would not have a hassle in finding one and Muriel would not have to wait for me. We parked on the first floor of the deck and took the elevator to Dr. Kretchmer's office. After we had removed our coats, the nurse checked Muriel's vital signs: weight (129 pounds), pulse (73), blood pressure (138/74), temperature (97.8°), and the oxygen in her system was determined to be at 99–100% with the Escort. In talking with Dr. Kretchmer, Muriel told him how she is faithfully using the Advair disks, the Atrovent, and albuterol inhalers, but is still suffering from shortness of breath when there is any exertion. She also mentioned the double vision. He decided to up her prednisone to 40 mg twice a day for five days, and then she will begin to taper off every five days until she is back to 10 mg per day. He also increased her Advair disk dosage. So two new prescriptions were provided when we left.

We had been home for about half an hour when Susan arrived to attend to Muriel. Her vital signs were again recorded: pulse (72), blood pressure (136/74), and respirations (24). As might be expected, the pulse and blood pressure were almost identical. I am happy for Muriel that all those who attend her have taken such great care of her. After Susan had examined Muriel with her stethoscope she said, "Your heart and lungs appear to be okay."

"I got the cane you had delivered, but I feel more comfortable leaning on Keith or using the furniture and walls as I move around the house."

"You can keep it in case you change your mind about using it."

"I saw Dr. Kretchmer today and he increased my prednisone, so it is a case of 'wait and see what happens' from this new dosage."

"What are your current pain levels?"

"It's a one for both my back and my ribs."

"So we don't need to change the medications?"

"Not at this time."

Mark, Cathy, and the family arrived just as Susan was finishing up, so everybody got introduced to Muriel's visiting nurse. I had put a roast in the oven after we had gotten home, and then made mashed potatoes and gravy along with green beans for dinner. For a moment I thought Mark was going to eat all of the roast. What amazed me more, he still had room for the pie I made. They kept Muriel company while I went to combined choir practice. When I returned, Mark and his family departed. I was glad to tuck Muriel in for the night and head for bed.

Wednesday, March 19, 2003

After I exercised this morning I took the two prescriptions from Dr. Kretchmer to CVS to be filled, and while I was at the drugstore I picked up a box of note cards for Muriel. Since she had gotten her diagnosis of three to six months, people from the congregation have been visiting her and sending her cards and notes. No matter how the empathy was conveyed, Muriel responded by writing a personal note to each of the individuals or couples. Many of the people told me they in turn were uplifted by such a kind gesture.

Mark, Cathy, and the girls arrived a little after lunch and we just sat around and talked. Because we are in the Lenten season, dinners are being held at the church before services, so we all trooped over there for dinner and then stayed for the Lenten service. It also afforded us an opportunity to show off two of our grandchildren and for Mark to talk with several individuals who were his contemporaries. When church was over, Mark and his family returned home with us. They planned to begin their two-day journey back to Texas in the morning and it was time to say goodbye. We gathered in the family room and Meagan and Emma expressed their love for Oma with hugs and tears. Cathy too gave Muriel a big hug and bid her goodbye. Mark, who had a special relationship with his mother, held her the longest with tears flowing down his cheeks, saying a special goodbye and promising to be one of the readers at her memorial service. We walked silently to the front door and they departed.

Friday, March 21, 2003

The Lincare man came this morning to refill Muriel's liquid oxygen container. He also dropped off two new cannulas for Muriel. The problem is that they get clogged and there is no way to clean them out, so one is for immediate use and one is for future use. These had ear protectors to prevent rubbing on the backside of the ear as the tubing is wrapped around to hold the cannula in place. I helped Muriel shower and wash her hair. Muriel generally weighed herself every day but doing so took energy, so she was inclined to do it just on the days she showered. The scale showed 125 pounds, down a little but not where she would like it. Susan arrived at 3:30 for her biweekly visit. She checked her pulse (88), blood pressure (142/84), and respirations (24). After Susan had checked her heart and lungs, Muriel said, "I am still having a problem with shortness of breath, especially with exertion, like taking a shower."

"I'd be happy to send in a home health assistant."

"No, not until I can no longer shower on my own."

Current pain levels for her back and ribs were at level one, so it was agreed that the medications can remain the same.

Tuesday, March 25, 2003

We spent the morning in the family room, and in the afternoon Muriel requested the comfort of her waterbed so we worked our way back upstairs. She ate her late lunch in bed, and since sitting upright in the waterbed was less stable than a chair, I fed her. That worked out very well and allowed us to determine that as she continues to deteriorate I will be able to nourish her. For one of the few times since she has been coming, Susan found Muriel in bed. I got her a chair next to the bed and she was her usual efficient self. Vital signs were taken: pulse (80), blood pressure (114/68), and respirations (24). She listened to her heart and lungs and then asked Muriel, "What are your pain levels today?"

"My back is a one and my ribs are a zero."

"It looks like your medications are under control. Do you have any other concerns today?"

"A member of my support group has cancer again, after not having any occurrence in the five years since she had breast cancer. I'm concerned she is going to end up like me, but facing death at a much younger age."

"All you can do is be positive when you are around her and give her as much emotional support as you can."

"When I was given my prognosis, I knew it would come sooner or later, but after Keith and I had a good cry it just became another bump in the road on what has become my adventure. I feel blessed to be experiencing this part of my life."

"Not everyone is as strong as you are, Muriel, or has the spiritual base that you have. You also get wonderful support from your husband and all the members of your church. Remember all of those cards you received? Send her a card to let her know you are thinking about her."

"You're right. I can certainly do that and I can always pray."

Friday, March 28, 2003

It was late afternoon when Susan arrived today, but no matter when she comes she is a welcome ray of sunshine. It is sometimes difficult to determine which of the two, Muriel or Susan, has a more positive attitude. It can be said that Susan, much like the oncology personnel in Dr. Koenig's office who deal with cancer patients day in and day out, are truly angels of mercy. Patients place great trust in them for the skills they possess and the counsel they provide. Muriel's vital signs were taken: pulse (84), blood pressure (124/72), and respirations (24). Her lungs were clear and her heart was at a regular rate and rhythm. She reported that her current pain levels were at a one for both her back and ribs.

Muriel seemed to be talkative after dinner tonight, and after a brief discussion regarding the visits of our children we got into reminiscing about our days at the university when we shared an office. To do so was rather unusual, as Muriel was in the English Department in the College of Arts and Sciences and I was a member of the Management Department in the College of Business Administration (CBA). However, there was some logic to this situation. Muriel was the copy editor for the *Akron Business and Economic Review*, a quarterly publication of the CBA, and she also edited articles for the business professors prior to sending them out for review and publication.

It all began in very tight quarters in Leigh Hall where we shared a single desk. From there we moved to Kolbe Hall where I had a much larger office so Muriel was able to have her own desk. After Kolbe Hall the CBA moved to a brand-new building across the tracks in downtown Akron where she had her own office right next to mine. People often wondered how we could spend time at home together and then "go to work" and spend more time together. However, it was not a problem for us as we enjoyed each other's company. Our conversation culminated in a discussion of the fire that was set in our office in Kolbe Hall. We are still speculating as to whether it was one of her students or one of mine, as there was no specific outcome of the fire department's investigation except to judge that it was a random occurrence. However, to us, the selection of the middle office on one side of the hall on the second floor of the building does not seem to be random.

Tuesday, April 1, 2003

I exercised this morning and then made a batch of muffins. At this stage Muriel's lunch, or should we say late breakfast, is a muffin and the fruit mix I have been making. The last time Sue d'Amico came to visit Muriel she brought along a baby monitoring system that she had used with her last child. Muriel has the microphone portion by her bed and I have the receiver wherever I am located, which could be in the family room, the basement, or, in the evening, on my nightstand. Muriel has had to get used to the fact that I do not instantly appear when she calls, particularly if I am in the basement. So in the morning I generally wait for her to "page" me and then I go up to assist wherever I can and help her to come downstairs for the day. Sometimes she will shower and dress and other times she will spend the day in her pajamas and robe. It is generally midmorning and after her cup of coffee and her pills that she will have her first meal of the day. After eating she might nap or watch a movie or we might talk a little.

Shirley Hayes, the hospice pain specialist, was in this afternoon to make an overall assessment of Muriel's pain situation. She took Muriel's vital signs: pulse (80), blood pressure (146/76), and respirations (20). "On a scale of zero to ten, what are the pain levels for your back and your ribs?" Shirley asked.

"Right now my back is a zero and my ribs are a two, although it is probably closer to one. As you know, I'm on a 12-hour regimen for my pain medications, so I took a dose just before you came."

"I see you are still on oxygen. I heard a little wheeze when I listened to your lungs. How is your breathing in general?"

"I bump my oxygen to five liters per minute when I take a shower and when I move from downstairs to upstairs, which is a real chore. I have been using the Advair disks and the Atrovent and albuterol inhalers on a regular basis to support my breathing. I think the prednisone also provides some aid in breathing. I have been on 10 mg twice a day, but starting tomorrow I will reduce it to 10 mg once a day."

"You're certainly doing all of the right things. However, I would like you to go on a nebulizer. I will have one delivered to your home this afternoon."

I chimed in, "What's a nebulizer?"

"It is designed to provide relief for one's breathing by creating a moist mist which is much better than the dry air we normally breathe. Are you still experiencing double vision?"

"Only in my left eye and it seems to be improving."

"How are you moving these days?"

"First, I don't really do much moving, as we use the wheelchair in the house as well as outside. However, on Saturday we are going to hear the Akron Symphony. Keith will deliver me to our seat area and then I will walk to my seat with his support and with the use of the railing. He also carries my oxygen at those times. Generally I get around pretty well with the help of the furniture and Keith. My real difficulty is the breathing when I expend any energy."

"It sounds like you're doing really well."

"I'm still on my adventure and God has blessed me with this new experience, and I am trying to make the most of it. I have great support from members of my church and my many friends. My only concern is the burden I place on Keith to care for me. He's doing everything!"

"That's because I love you," I said.

Muriel was pretty hyped up after Shirley left, so we sat and talked. Most of the talking we do these days is a recollection of earlier times, and today we talked about the first time she came to visit me on the farm in Hamlin, New York when I had returned from my freshman year at Clarkson University. I had a day job at Eastman Kodak Company and several evenings a week I washed dishes at the Lyon's Den, a bowling establishment and eatery. However, while she was up from New Jersey I limited my evening working hours. "Do you remember the night we went to the Genesee Park Inn?"

Muriel smiled. "The GPI? That was quite a night. I think we danced to Johnny Mathis the whole evening."

"That was when 'The Twelfth of Never' became an all-time favorite. I don't think we could really call it dancing. The place was so crowded we just stood in one spot and swayed to the music. Okay, what was the next song we added to our trilogy of pop songs?"

"It was Kenny Rogers' rendition of 'Through the Years,' and it was solidified when we received a recorded message from that Marriage Encounter team couple from Columbus."

"Yes, that was Wayne and Robin Ferne."

"You remember their names?"

"That's why I get paid the big money. If you recall, they sent us a thank-you tape for giving them the opportunity to be part of our presenting team that weekend. I guess since you included the trilogy in your memorial service, you know the last one also."

Muriel began to tear up as she said, "Henry Mancini's 'Softly as I Leave You.'"

Seeing her begin to cry I, too, had tears stream down my cheeks. I moved from my chair to a stool in front of Muriel so we could embrace and hold each other, because the time was coming when it truly would be "Softly as I Leave You." I really think that I am blessed to be able to mourn Muriel's passing while she is still alive through the sharing of incidences from our time together. There is a certain cleansing effect and it just draws us closer together.

Wednesday, April 2, 2003

We continue to use the scale that we established earlier regarding Muriel's pain levels. However, she had transitioned from OxyIR to MSIR for immediate relief. It seems to me that with the change to MSIR, she is using more capsules toward the end of the OxyContin cycle, and often in between. We went to church this evening, and we arrived early so we could attend the dinner. There were many well-wishers who came by to talk with Muriel. Sally Haller and Shirley Williams made a date to see her on Thursday. The Chorale sang for the service with Muriel in attendance, but under its de facto leader, Susan. Muriel continues to inspire me in the way she is proceeding on this adventure. It is sometimes hard to fathom the mental toughness that she exhibits as she works her way through each day.

Saturday, April 5, 2003

I exercised early this morning and then helped Muriel get downstairs and settled in her La-Z-Boy recliner. We are now into the 4th month of the three to six month prognosis, and we have no way of knowing whether the end is near or whether Muriel's life will be prolonged beyond that time period. She just carries on very positively in her life. When people visit her, she responds with a note back to them a day or two after the visit. People tell me they can't believe that she had taken the time to respond to the visit, and in turn were uplifted. Today, she wanted to talk about her 50th birthday bash and how pleased she had been about the whole day. Our conversation hopped and skipped around, so I will provide you the flavor of that day from the letter Muriel wrote to her mother.

Dear Mom,

Received your letter and was glad to hear the ring arrived safely. All is well here, although I'm still recovering from my 50th birthday. I don't think I've ever experienced a birthday, much less a day, that comes even close.

The day began for me at seven o'clock when I came downstairs to find a beautiful big candle burning and a birthday card on the kitchen table. The candle is soft pastel diagonal bands that subtly blend into each other. Keith knows how I love candles, and I find it so relaxing to light it and watch it for a while when I am taking a break.

A little before ten o'clock Keith left for the university to meet with another prof with whom he is doing some research. Not more than five minutes after he left—he had planned it that way—there was a knock on the door. It turned out to be the florist. Her little girl came in first with a straw flower arrangement that was a gift from a former student. The vase, which is white with an iris on it, matches our bedroom drapes and comforter beautifully, so I have the arrangement on my desk in there. Then Heidi (the florist) came in with an arrangement of fifty yellow roses! It was overwhelming! Yellow roses have always been my favorite flower, and since they were the first flowers Keith ever gave me before we were married, they have always been especially meaningful. The scent permeated the entire downstairs. After a week they are still doing well, although a few are on their last legs—or stems or petals or whatever.

It was a rather gloomy day as far as the weather was concerned—overcast with rain threatening—and as we headed for lunch time (Keith was home by now but I didn't plan lunch as I knew we were going out for dinner—about the only thing I did know about that day!) I began to feel sleepy. I didn't want to be tired when we went out in the evening, so I thought I would take a nap but decided to wait until the mail came, which is usually a little after noon. The mail arrived and I got some more birthday cards, a letter from the mayor of Munroe Falls issuing a proclamation for my birthday, and a newspaper with the headline "Muriel Klafehn Reaches Fiftieth Year!" Keith had arranged for both of those and had also made sure they would come in the mail on my birthday.

By this time it was after one o'clock and I went upstairs to bed. I read for a while and then tried to sleep but had some difficulty because of all the excitement. Somewhere around two I dozed off until almost three-thirty. When I came downstairs, Keith said he had to meet with the graduate student whom he had arranged with to teach his classes that night so we could go out on my birthday and not the day after. I found out later that wasn't where he went! Anyway, after he left I went upstairs to shower. I happened to glance out the bathroom window, which faces the front of the house, and saw blurry lights and a fuzzy arrow. I didn't have my glasses on at the time, so I went to get them and looked out the window again. There, parked on our front lawn, was a big electric sign all lit up. On one side it said "Lo and Behold Mom is 50 Years Old" and the other side read "Honk—Mom is 50 Years Old." Mark had arranged for it and it had been delivered while I was sleeping! Then I began to notice all the honks as people drove by the house. Kids would ride by on bicycles and yell "honk, honk, beep, beep." It was fun, and since the sign wasn't picked up until the next evening, I had a second day of honks.

I finally showered and then had a cup of coffee before getting dressed for dinner. I was sitting in the kitchen and Keith was in the family room having come back from his "meeting." About four-thirty there was a knock on the door. I had just my terry robe on, so I looked in at Keith, but he said I could get it. It was the man from UPS with a big package. (Having seen the sign on the lawn—who could miss it—he said he felt he should sing "Happy Birthday.") I brought the package inside and opened it. On the top was another card from Keith and inside the box were five bags of barbecued potato chips! I sat right down on the floor and laughed until the tears ran and my sides ached. You see, every once in a while, usually late at night, I'll get a craving for potato chips, and then dear Keith will drive around looking for a store that's open. It's become a family joke. So Keith arranged to have the five bags of chips—one for each ten years—delivered on my birthday.

By now I wondered what else could happen and figured nothing else could. Except, of course, going out to dinner. Keith had made reservations for six-thirty at the Triple Crown, a lovely restaurant just down the road from us. We had taken Mark there for his birthday last December. We had a delicious dinner, going all out. First we had a drink—I had a vodka martini and Keith had a Bloody Mary (he says he likes the celery)—and Keith read me his two-page birthday poem he wrote. More tears! I had a shrimp cocktail, salad, and Veal Florentine with a glass of White Zinfandel. Keith had herring, salad, scallops, and Chablis. With our coffee I had a B & B and Keith had a Crème de Cocoa. While I was savoring all this, all of a sudden a waitress came to the table with a birthday cake, and she and two other waitresses sang "Happy Birthday." There was a group at the table near us, and one of the men peeked over at the cake, which had "Happy 50th Birthday Muriel" on it. He said if they had known it was my 50th birthday they would have sung too. So then all the people at that table sang "Happy Birthday."

We left the restaurant a little after eight o'clock, and I anticipated coming home, putting on my comfortable robe, and watching Hitchcock's "Vertigo" on the movie channel. When I walked into the kitchen something didn't seem right. *Everything was dark, whereas we usually leave the light on over the stove when we go out at night. I flipped on the switch for the ceiling light and just stood there staring at the kitchen counters. They were cluttered with bottles, a cooler, cups, etc. I <u>knew</u> they had been cleared off before we left! Then came the shout of "Surprise" from the dark of the family room, and it seemed as if people were materializing out of every nook and cranny.*

All of this, from the time I walked into the kitchen until the "surprise," was just a matter of seconds, but in my dazed state it seemed to be happening in slow motion. My first surprise party! There were friends from church, from Marriage Encounter, and from the university. They had all arrived just a little after we had left for the restaurant and had a buffet dinner Keith had planned and provided. That was the reason for his "meeting" that afternoon. He had gone to pick up the food, etc. and delivered it at a friend's house who then brought it all over to our place. Keith got teased about his signal for our arrival home. He had told everyone he would honk the car horn as we pulled into the driveway, which wouldn't have been suspicious as he sometimes accidentally hits the horn making the turn. However, with Mark's sign out front, honking had been going on all evening!

I had another birthday cake and we had cake and champagne and presents. Among others, I got a thirty-dollar gift certificate to Waldenbooks. The givers of that gift certainly know me well and I anticipate browsing and getting books like the proverbial child in the candy store. Another thoughtful gift was a gift certificate to Blossom Music Center where the Cleveland Orchestra has their summer concerts. Once when Richard and Judith were here we took them there.

The party broke up about midnight as the next day was a working day. I think Mark was the last to leave. I missed not having Kay there, but she did call around nine o'clock. Keith told me later that he had debated flying her here for the occasion, but that didn't work out as she had just started work at her new job the day before. When everyone was gone, Keith said there was still more and asked me to make myself comfortable in the family room. Then he got the tape recorder and a handful of tapes and for about two hours we listened to birthday messages from friends around the country—from Tacoma, Washington to Washington, D.C., and from St. Paul, Minnesota to Houston, Texas. Even friends in Canada were included. It was an overwhelming experience, filled with laughter and tears, listening to voices I hadn't heard for a while and knowing that all these people cared enough to take the time to tape the messages, which included original poems, all sorts of musical renditions, and lots of shared memories. It was just as overwhelming to discover that Keith had been planning this day for six months, starting in December right after Christmas.

The very last message on the tape was from Keith, indicating that there was one last surprise for me. I didn't know what else there could possibly be and whether my heart could stand another surprise. I teased him, saying that now I knew why he had increased my life insurance as much <u>before</u> my birthday! He went upstairs again and came down with another card and a large jeweler's box. Inside was a black velvety case, and when I opened that I found a 23-inch string of matched cultured pearls! I thought I had died and gone to heaven. I have always wanted, even coveted, a set of real pearls and now I had them. Fortunately Keith had them appraised and insured before he gave them to me or I would have been afraid to wear them as they are valued at $950.00.

We finally got to bed in the wee hours of the morning. I told Keith that I didn't need another birthday for the rest of my life as nothing could top this one. He said that maybe now he could sleep—as apparently he got more and more nervous the closer it got to my birthday wondering whether all would go well and being concerned about timing. It all went perfectly, I never suspected any of it and my dear husband is the ultimate prince among men.

Sorry this is so long, but I wanted to share "my day" with you.
Much love,
Muriel

We of course did not discuss the birthday in quite the detail that is given above, but many of the items were discussed and we did get out the tapes and listen to them again. As noted in the letter we laughed and cried, probably a little more than we did the first time we heard them. For Muriel it may be the last time she hears many of those voices.

I helped Muriel take a shower and get dressed. While she primped I got our dinner started. While that was underway I filled the portable oxygen tank and then changed clothes. I prepared plates for each of us and we ate off our usual TV trays while watching the news. The dishes went in the dishwasher and then we drove to E. J. Thomas Hall to hear a subscription concert by the Akron Symphony Orchestra. We arrived in plenty of time, parked the wheelchair outside the auditorium, and made our way to our regular seats. Ya-Hui Wang had opened with Edvard Grieg's *Peer Gynt* Suite No. 1, Op. 46. It is a popular piece in the repertoire of many orchestras and I thought it was well-played. The selection just before intermission featured the horn section of the orchestra playing Schumann's *Konzertstück for Four Horns* in F Major, Op. 86. The four horns did a marvelous job, and it was great that the music director chose a piece that would enable them to be highlighted.

The final piece played after intermission was Scriabin's Symphony No. 2 in C Minor, Op. 29. Considering our afternoon tear fest and an evening of beautiful music, we went home in a euphoric state.

Tuesday, April 8, 2003

We were expecting a visit from Susan Slagle from VNS today, but instead welcomed Pamela Caldwell. With all that has transpired during this adventure, you learn to go with the flow. She began with the usual vital signs: pulse (80), blood pressure (112/70), and respirations (22). She used her stethoscope and listened to Muriel's heart and her breathing. Pain levels were checked, currently at one for both her back and ribs. Muriel described her pain as a slight burning/stinging most of the time, and then increasing to a sharp localized pain. That was when she usually took the MSIR capsules according to our sliding scale. I told Pam that we are getting low on OxyContin. She said she would call Dr. Koenig's office and have it renewed. Unlike Susan, who chitchats with us, Pam was gone in 20 minutes.

An interesting sidebar that arose today came about through a call from Ed Celentano. He is the class agent for Muriel's graduating class at Montclair State in New Jersey, who is organizing a 50th college reunion. Muriel informed him all about her adventure and that, in a sense, she is waiting to die. He was extremely empathetic to her situation, and I think she was very glad to have an opportunity to share her plight with a complete stranger. The bottom line is Muriel will not be able to attend the reunion. I wonder what thoughts Ed had after speaking with Muriel.

Saturday, April 12, 2003

Last night we went to Ohio Ballet at the Akron Civic Theatre. Muriel enjoyed the opportunity to get out and, as she put it, act normal, or at least as normal as one can be while in a wheelchair and using oxygen.

Susan was back from her one-day hiatus and we were happy to see her smiling face and to participate in the constant interaction that she provides. Muriel's vital signs were recorded: pulse (88), blood pressure (120/64), and respirations (24). Muriel offered pain levels. "It's a one for my back and a one for my ribs."

"Do your regular meds meet your needs? You know you can change them if you are having any difficulty."

"I think the medications are okay, but what concerns me right now is my ability to stay awake in the evening. I have no idea that my eyes are closing, and before I know it, I have slept for thirty minutes to an hour.

I often sleep late in the morning, and that's great, but I don't like what is happening in the evening."

"First of all, you have to realize that all the medication you are taking is, in a sense, numbing your system. In addition, the disease itself is beginning to take a toll on your body. You look fine to me. However, if falling asleep is a real problem we can add Ritalin to your meds."

"I never have trouble sleeping or falling asleep, but I would like to stay awake in the evening. I'm scheduled to see Dr. Koenig on Tuesday. I'll discuss it with him."

"It's a pleasure to come visit you, Muriel, because you just refuse to give in."

When Susan finished with Muriel, I walked with her to the front door and thanked her for all of her help. She replied, "It really is my pleasure. She's an inspiration." She paused, then added, "You're an inspiration as well, Keith. Muriel's fortunate for all of the support you give to her."

"Muriel is so positive, it's a privilege to care for her."

Tuesday, April 15, 2003

In addition to being income tax day, we had two appointments today, one at 2:00 with Dr. Koenig, and at 3:00 we were to see Dr. Kretchmer. So after lunch I filled Muriel's portable oxygen tank and we set off for the physician's office building for the scheduled appointments. We have found that afternoon appointments enable us to get in to see the doctor more readily, and such was the case today. Muriel was weighed (135¼ pounds) and her blood pressure was taken (136/70). I think Dr. Koenig was pleased to see how well Muriel is doing. They talked about pain management and whether or not she thinks things are under control. Muriel said, "I think the pain is under control, but I am concerned about falling asleep without notice."

Much like Susan had done, Dr. Koenig expressed, "Your body is continuing to adjust to medication, and the progression of the disease also may cause you to involuntarily close your eyes and place your body in sleep mode. I could give you something to keep you awake, but I advise against it." Muriel yielded to his recommendation and agreed to stay the course for now.

I had brought the wheelchair, so we moved easily to Dr. Kretchmer's office. Muriel has greatly appreciated having a wheelchair since walking is such a chore and exacerbates her shortness of breath. Even when one is on oxygen, additional exertion causes undue stress to the respiration system. I know it is important that each doctor has his or her own set of vitals, but having just come from Dr. Koenig's office there seems to be a redundancy. Nevertheless, the following information was recorded at Dr. Kretchmer's office: weight (136½ pounds), blood pressure (144/82), pulse (78), temperature (96.2°), and oxygen saturation (99%). The conversation centered around the use of the prednisone. Muriel indicated that she had tapered off to 5 mg per day and then went back to 10 mg per day, helping her to feel better. He checked her airways and discussed the use of the inhalers she is on. He concluded that she should continue on the medications she is presently using and wishes to see her in one month. We worked our way back to the car and drove home.

Wednesday, April 16, 2003

Pastor Larry made a visit to Muriel today and apparently they had a delightful time, as laughter often emanated from the family room. Before he departed he gave us Communion together.

Thursday, April 17, 2003

Midafternoon I made a call to Dr. Koenig's office to ask for approval to increase the frequency of the dosage for the Valium Muriel is taking. The use of Valium is part of Muriel's overall pain relief regimen, and she wants to increase the frequency from every eight hours to every six hours. At just about 5:00, Christina Allison from hospice called. She let us know that Dr. Koenig had approved Muriel's request and she should start today. Muriel hopes that by altering the dosage of the Valium she will take fewer MSIR capsules.

We went to the Maundy Thursday church services in the evening as the Chorale was singing. It was a real chore for Muriel to get up the stairs to the balcony, and after we had gone to Communion together we found a seat in the nave for the rest of the service. Muriel received the well-wishes of many of the parishioners as they came by to hug her and express their concern for her. As is often the case, many of those people were bolstered by speaking with her.

Friday, April 18, 2003

Fred and Jean Mickelson visited Muriel today. Fred and Jean are a clergy couple, with whom we had done several weekends in Marriage Encounter. They are also a part of the M. E. team community, so they have been monitoring the progress of Muriel's disease and wanted to come and offer comfort and care. The four of us shared and reminisced about our weekends together, causing us to laugh and to shed tears. It may be the last time Fred and Jean see Muriel.

Susan arrived later in the afternoon with her little black bag and took Muriel's vital signs: pulse (88), blood pressure (120/70), and respirations (24). She listened to her heart and checked her lungs. "How are your pain levels today?"

"My back is a two and my ribs are a zero, but the pain in the area of the liver is a seven. I have been using more breakthrough medications over the last three days, and I want to have better control of the pain."

Susan called Dr. Koenig's office to suggest an increase in her dosage of OxyContin to a level of 160 mg every 12 hours. Karen Mascio, a nurse in Dr. Koenig's office, was the go-between and reported that they would fax a new prescription today to the CVS pharmacy to make that change. I picked up the new prescription in the evening and we will begin a new regimen of 160 mg of OxyContin every 12 hours.

Tuesday, April 22, 2003

In spite of the increase in OxyContin, we don't seem to be getting a handle on the pain, and Muriel has been using additional MSIR capsules to assuage the pain. So we were looking forward to the visit of the hospice nurse this afternoon. Karen Marshall arrived a little past 2:00 and took Muriel's vital signs: pulse (80), temperature (97.0°), blood pressure (140/90), and respirations (18). Next came the checking of her heart and lungs, and then an assessment of the pain levels. With the increase in the OxyContin Muriel has been having little problem with her back and ribs, but in the area of her liver she has been dealing with pains as high as nine on a scale of one to ten. Muriel indicated the current level was a seven. Karen called hospice and talked with Shirley Hayes, the pain specialist, and after consulting with Dr. Koenig, indicated that he was putting her on Decadron. Initially she is to take 8 mg and then will drop back to 4 mg every 12 hours.

Wednesday, April 23, 2003

After Muriel got up she was still having difficulty with pain, so I called hospice to talk with Shirley Hayes. She indicated she would call me back, and later in the afternoon she called and suggested that Muriel come to the hospice care center where she could be monitored more closely. After dinner, I put Muriel in the car and we drove to the care center in Fairlawn. We didn't know what to expect or how long Muriel will be there, but she was placed in a bed. She was hooked up to the internal oxygen system and given an intravenous shot which seemed to reduce her pain level. She seemed groggy and wanted to sleep, so I kissed her goodbye and headed home. I called both of our kids when I got home and shared with them the status of their mother. I also suggested that they do not plan on coming to visit Muriel as there is no scheduled date of death and I think it will be difficult for them to sit around in Ohio when their families and jobs are in Texas. I promised to keep them informed and call them on Sundays when I know they will both be home.

Thursday, April 24, 2003

After lunch I visited Muriel at the care center. I brought along something to eat so I could share dinner with her when the time came. I also brought along the book she has been reading, her crossword puzzle book, and a deck of cards that I think would help Muriel pass the time. While I was there Susan from VNS stopped in. "How is your pain now?"

"I don't know what they gave me when I first came in, but it sure took care of the pain. In fact, I get relief with each dose I request."

"You're an insider here, so what's happening?" I asked.

"I discussed the care plan and medication regime with Dr. Driscoll and she indicated that she has switched Muriel to MS Contin and is weaning her off the Neurontin."

"Is that better than the OxyContin?" I asked.

"No better, no worse. I think she just wants to make it so that the main medication and the breakthrough medication be the same."

Muriel said, "I think they gave me some Roxanol, a liquid morphine, but I didn't think it worked that well."

"From what I understand, Dr. Driscoll felt you were discussing pain caused by bone metastasis and not neuropathic pain."

"Well, I am happy to be at the care center because they seem to have a good handle on my pain."

"I am happy to hear that and I'll stop in again next week."

I thought to myself, *next week?* How long is she going to be here? Is she even going to come home from here? I had a chill as to the thought that maybe she won't get much past the three months in that three to six months prognosis.

Monday, April 28, 2003

I have been visiting Muriel each day, sometimes going in the morning, taking my lunch with me, and staying until just before dinner. Other days I go in after lunch and stay through dinner. The ladies of Fairlawn Lutheran Church provide chicken soup by the gallon for those persons visiting loved ones at the care center. So on days I have dinner with

Muriel, I have chicken soup and then stay until 8:00 or so. They seem to have gotten the medications regulated and she seems to be in less pain. However, one side effect of larger doses of a narcotic is the tendency to be more lethargic. She also seems to be having increasing difficulty breathing than with the pain management.

We were able to play Phase 10, but we did not complete any games because Muriel found it difficult to concentrate for long periods of time. Her great love of reading is also limited for the same reason. When she is lucid we talk. She again entreated for me to get on with my life after she was gone: "Go find a good woman and get married, you're too young to continue on by yourself," she says. Here she is dying, and she is concerned about my life after she is gone. Throughout this whole adventure she has been so positive and it has helped me to be optimistic about a full recovery, but that avenue seems to be closing. However, we both continue to pray for a miracle. True to her word, Susan stopped in again today to check on Muriel.

< 16 >
THE END IS CLOSE AT HAND

Friday, May 2, 2003

I had been notified yesterday during my visit that Muriel could come home today. So I eagerly arrived at the hospice care center midmorning with the intent of putting her in the car and returning home. She was dressed and appeared to be ready to go, but I sensed a reluctance to leave the security of the care center. They had taken great care of her, and after almost ten days there had to be the thought of whether or not that kind of care would continue. I reached over and took her hand as she sat in the wheelchair and said, "Muriel dear, I assure you, I can take care of you and provide for your needs, and if at any time you judge that my care is not adequate I will bring you back to the care center in a heartbeat."

"Okay then, wheel me to the car. The adventure will continue at 87 Oakhurst Drive."

I'm really not sure what I am getting myself into, but she trusts me. I wheeled her to the car, intent on doing my best to care for Muriel. As we turned to go, the discharge nurse said, "Muriel has been on a nebulizer while she's been here. A similar unit has been ordered through VNS and will be delivered to your home this afternoon. We also ordered a portable commode so Muriel could take care of necessities without having to walk to the bathroom, taxing her respiratory system."

"Thank you so very much for doing all of those things. I can under-stand why she wants to stay, you've taken such good care of her." I was also given a listing of her medications, together with the proper dosage and frequency, that I jealously guarded so I could prepare Muriel's medications for the day. A copy of this list is given below.

HOME MEDICATIONS INFORMATION

TYPE	DOSAGE	FREQUENCY
Decadron	12 mg	2x/day with food
Neurontin	200 mg	3x/day
Multivitamin		One each day
Dulcolax	5 mg tabs	1 a.m. and 1 p.m.
Senocot	2 tablets	1 a.m. and 1 p.m.
Protonix	40 mg	Once per day
Valium	2.5 mg	8 a.m. • 4 p.m. • 12 a.m.
Nasonex	2 puffs/nostril	Each day
Roxanol	40-100 mg	Every hour as needed
Allegra	60 mg	Breakfast & bedtime
MS Contin	300 mg	8 a.m. • 4 p.m. • 12 a.m.
Prozac	10 mg	12 a.m.
Synthroid	50 mcg	Every morning
Viokase	16 mg	Three tabs with meals
Zinc		One tab each day
Selenium	100 mcg	One tab each day
Albuterol	2.5 mg	Every four hours when awake
Atrovent	5 mg	Every four hours when awake

The last two items on the list are used with the nebulizer. Muriel was taking many of the medications on the list before she went to the hospice care center. The basic changes were the MS Contin at 300 mg and the use of Roxanol, a liquid morphine to be used for breakthrough pain. Prior to going to the care center she had been taking 160 mg of OxyContin and was using MSIR for breakthrough pain. After we got home and Muriel was settled into her recliner, I made some soup for rf

gmen ye="head_ig>IT WAS A PRIVILEGE TO CARE FOR HER

her lunch. We used a towel for a bib and I fed her, as it seemed much easier than having her dribble the soup down the front of her due to an unsteady hand. I had begun feeding her while she was at the care center, so it is a logical extension. She dozed part of the afternoon and then I fed her dinner. While I was feeding her dinner I suggested, "Let's set up a scale for using Roxanol as we had done for the MSIR."

Perhaps she had been thinking about it also as she quickly responded, "At a zero or one, I judge that there is no need to take any. A persistent three or four, I'd suggest 40 cc, five or six probably 60 cc, seven or eight will be 80 cc, and if it reaches the nine or ten range we will use 100 cc."

"Sounds good to me. So when appropriate, you give the pain level and I will wield the syringe."

I managed to get her upstairs in the early evening and set up the nebulizer, which we had used in the afternoon just before dinner. After her treatment she again dozed and I returned downstairs. We still have the communication system intact, so she knows if she needs me she just has to speak into the microphone and I will be right up. She did call me at about 10:30 as the effects of the 4:00 MS Contin dosage began to wear off, and I gave her some Roxanol. I made the judgment that in the short period of time we were home she was confident that I could adequately care for her. Right away she began with the *You need to play bridge* and *You need to play golf* requests. It was the age-old plea that my life should be normal even if hers is not. She tried again saying, "Lois Jenkins would probably be happy to come in and sit with me if she were not working."

"Yes my dear, I know, and we will do that. We will also investigate the use of home health care with Susan the next time she comes."

Saturday, May 3, 2003

The main accomplishment for the day was assisting Muriel to take a bath. Using the flexible hose extension while seated on the blue plastic stool placed in the middle of the tub, Muriel can sit and wash and rinse herself as well as being able to shampoo and rinse her hair. However, now that she is a little weaker and doesn't have as much energy to expend, I have become responsible for washing and rinsing her hair. The shower and tub area is enclosed with sliding doors so it is easy to lean in and do her hair without any problems.

Monday, May 5, 2003

I attended church by myself yesterday and had public prayers of thanksgiving offered on Muriel's behalf for the regulation of her pain. Muriel decided to stay in bed this morning so I provided her with

247

breakfast in bed. I said, "It is a little difficult trying to give you a sip of coffee without giving you too big a slug. I think we should get one of those child cups with the spout and then you could give yourself sips."

"Sounds like a good idea to me."

"Hey, I'm just yanking your chain." After we had a good laugh she said, "I still think it's a good idea, my own sippy cup."

Robin Graham, from Muriel's support group, was in to visit later in the morning and the three of us sat around and chatted. Robin asked, "Where does Muriel have her TV?" She was appalled to find out that we have only one TV in the house. So I said, "Here's my credit card. Go to Walmart and get us a brand new TV that could play tapes as well." About 20 minutes later she was back with a 21-inch TV that will sit nicely right on the bookcase in front of Muriel's bed. I thanked her and said, "Robin you are to be commended for bringing us into the modern world with more than one television in our house." Later in the day, I called Time Warner to have someone come out and install the cable in the bedroom so the TV could be hooked up to the cable. They will come out in a few days. Muriel will watch videos, or perhaps sleep through videos, until the cable is hooked up.

This afternoon Susan made her first visit since Muriel has come home from the care center and greeted her in the bedroom. "Hello there girl, how are you doing?"

"I've seen better days, but I'm happy to be home with my sweetheart taking care of me."

"I see he got you a new TV."

"Yes, he sent my friend Robin from my support group to Walmart to get it this morning."

At that point, I jumped in and asked, "What can you tell me about getting home health care?"

"I'll have someone give you a call." She then proceeded to examine Muriel. A check of the vital signs indicated pulse (88), blood pressure (160/90), and respirations (28). She then listened to Muriel's heart and lungs and reported that everything was in order. "What are your current pain levels?"

"They are quite low. After we got home, Keith and I worked out a sliding scale for using Roxanol for breakthrough pain in a similar manner to the use of the MSIR."

"You wanted to have your pain controlled at a two to three level. Apparently that is happening."

"So far, so good."

When I walked Susan downstairs, she said, "I think Muriel looks a little lethargic, but that is understandable considering all the medication she is taking."

I don't know if she was trying to tell me that Muriel is in the throes of the dying process, but I put it out of my head for the moment.

Wednesday, May 7, 2003

I was due to play golf this morning and Lois Jenkins had agreed to come and sit with Muriel. Since she is an RN, I knew Muriel was in good hands. She is still serving as Muriel's Stephen Minister, so that is even better. All went well while I was out. Lois had given her breakfast and run the nebulizer to assist her in her breathing. Midmorning Lois had received a call from Karla Maple about home health care and she suggested that she call me back later. I spoke with Karla later in the day and suggested she drop by, as Muriel wanted to meet her. Karla arrived at 3:00 and met Muriel. She answered all of Muriel's questions concerning what a home health care aide does and offered her a foot massage, a hand massage, or a back rub, all of which Muriel declined. As Karla departed she said, "Maybe next time."

Friday, May 9, 2003

I exercised this morning before Muriel stirred and was all set to provide her with breakfast and her complement of medications when she awoke. I also hooked up the nebulizer, which we have been running every four hours when Muriel is awake. After lunch Kristen Spetich, a home health care aide, came by. She gave Muriel a sponge bath in bed, helped her with her hair, and rubbed her all over with lotion. She also helped her to get dressed. After Kristen had left, I helped Muriel get downstairs and into her La-Z-Boy recliner. When she was squared away, she said, "It's nice to have a home health care aide."

"See, never look a gift horse in the mouth."

Susan arrived at 3:45 and greeted Muriel in the family room. Susan checked Muriel's vital signs: pulse (84), blood pressure (156/80), and respirations (28). On checking her heart and lungs she said, "I detect some wheezing similar to what you had experienced at the care center."

"Is that a problem?" I asked.

"I don't think so, but we want to keep track of it. What are your pain levels Muriel?"

She mumbled something and Susan said, "I didn't hear that."

"I'm out of it too much," she stammered.

I said, "They are probably zero or one or she would let us know. I think she needs a lot of time to answer questions, as it is increasingly difficult for her to process things. She stopped journaling some time ago."

Susan and I carried on the conversation almost as if Muriel was not there. Susan said, "I noticed she now seems to have uncontrollable movements in both of her hands."

"Yes, and as a result I am feeding her all of the time now."

Muriel was in fact listening though, as she stumblingly stated, "It gives us a time together for sharing and devotions."

"However, she no longer seems to worry about sleeping too much," I offered.

Before she departed, Susan said, "Call the care center or Dr. Koenig if you see any significant changes."

Muriel has the TV on most of the day, but often falls asleep while it is on. She requests videos, which I gladly get and put into the machine only to find that she dozed off during part of the movie. So I rewind it to the point where she fell asleep, if she remembers, and play it from there. We have always had daily devotions but had generally done them separately. Now we're having our devotions together, as I can do all of the readings that are appropriate. One of the prayers she has been using is entitled "On Dying." It is a wonderful prayer, and I read it to her every morning and every evening. As the need arises I help her to get out of bed and use the portable commode, which is placed right next to the bed. Meals represent the major time when we have the opportunity to share and have meaningful exchanges.

Tuesday, May 13, 2003

Karla Maple was in yesterday to give Muriel a sponge bath in bed and to help her with other ablutions. She also helped her to get dressed for the afternoon so she could come downstairs. Today it was my turn to help Muriel get her teeth brushed, her hair combed, her body washed, and get her dressed, because she wanted to be downstairs when Susan came. When Susan arrived she was surprised to find Muriel in the family room. First came the vital signs: pulse (108), blood pressure (130/76), and respirations (28). She listened to her heart and lungs and jokingly said, "I heard some good crackles. What are your pain levels today?"

"Everything is under control and has been for the last three days," Muriel offered.

I added, "I think we need a renewal of the MS Contin."

"I'll call Dr. Koenig's office and have that taken care of."

Muriel slurred out the words, "Keith is feeding me all my meals and I really enjoy those quiet periods with him."

"That way I don't have to change the bed linens after each meal," I humorously posited.

Muriel continued haltingly, "I seem to be spending most of the time sleeping, but I have managed to get downstairs once a day for two to three hours. Lately I have been having nosebleeds."

"I think if you use a water-soluble gel in your nose applied with a cotton tipped applicator you will find some relief."

Wednesday, May 14, 2003

I continue to be the secretary of the Stow Senior Men's Golf League and today was a scheduled day of play. I had made arrangements to have a home health care aide for the day and Jackie Reiff, a University of Akron nursing student, arrived at 8:00 to care for Muriel. I had awakened Muriel for her morning medications and fed her breakfast. I advised Jackie of where she could find Muriel's lunch and bade her goodbye. I returned at 2:30 and Jackie informed me she had given Muriel lunch and had shampooed and brushed her hair.

When I had finished feeding Muriel tonight and gotten everything cleaned up she said, "Get the gold chain in the center drawer of my jewelry box please." I complied. "Now, I'd like the pendant you gave me that was etched with 'Soaring Above the Storm.'" I again did as she requested. "Please put the pendant on the chain." So I undid the clasp and put the pendant on the chain. I was about to reclasp the chain when she touched my arm, and as I looked to her in the bed she took off her wedding band and motioned for me to put it on the chain also. Then I reclasped the chain and brought it to her, as I thought she wanted it around her neck. However, she said, "Bend down," and then proceeded to put the chain over my head. I was blown away and tears welled up in my eyes and gushed down my cheeks. It was her way of saying goodbye and that she was ready to die. With my help she had done everything she wanted to do. I sat on the edge of the bed and held her close. I whispered in her ear, "I love you so very much and will miss you greatly." We both cried, knowing that our life together as a couple is drawing to a close.

Thursday, May 15, 2003

I awakened her with a cup of coffee this morning, and she actually seemed upset that she hadn't died last night after giving me her ring. I said, "Welcome to a new day. It's time to take your morning pills and if you do that I will give you breakfast." She took her medications and I returned with a muffin to accompany her coffee. She knew that it was Thursday and asked, "Are you playing bridge today?" Knowing her concern for me not missing out on my activities I assured her, saying "I am playing bridge this afternoon." Jackie, the home health care aide, arrived at 11:00 and gave her lunch, but according to Jackie's report Muriel refused all other services. Jackie said she just seemed tired and wanted to rest.

Friday, May 16, 2003

Our regular Susan was on vacation and Suzanne Hamrick, who was covering for her, arrived at 11:20. Muriel was still upstairs in bed so I brought Suzanne upstairs to examine her. The vitals signs showed an increase in her pulse reading (110) with the blood pressure at a decent level (130/82) and respirations normal (28). Muriel continues on the 300 mg of MS Contin three times a day and it is doing a great job of covering her pain. She has not used any breakthrough medication for some time. So all of the pain levels were at a zero. She continues to have a little rattle in her breathing, and it is labored according to Suzanne's report, but her heart still seems to be going strong. Suzanne shared with me, "Muriel's overall mental capacity is deteriorating, as she needs prompting to respond to questions."

"I have seen that also as we talk during mealtime."

After Suzanne had left, I just sat by the bed and held Muriel's hand as she drifted in and out of sleep. I think she knew that I needed to get away to play golf and to play bridge, because it is so gut-wrenching to see the woman I love deteriorate right before my eyes.

Saturday, May 17, 2003

Muriel wanted to have a shower today, so I got her out of bed and into the tub and positioned her on the stool. I soaped her all over and she seemed to enjoy the water cascading on her body. I thoroughly washed her hair and then dried her off and put her in fresh pajamas. Afterward, I changed the sheets on the bed so she would have a nice clean place to rest.

Muriel was alert after the stimulation of the shower and we began chatting, which led to more reminiscing. On a Marriage Encounter weekend we did in Detroit we met a couple who had just had a wonderful experience on their weekend. They shared with us at the end of the weekend that they had a cabin on the Au Sable River in Grayling, Michigan and that we were welcomed to use it anytime for as long as we wanted. So we took them up on their offer and spent a week at the cabin renewing our relationship and enjoying the great outdoors.

One of those days we took a 25-mile canoe trip. Neither of us had canoed before and after four complete 360° turns we finally got the hang of it. The current was swift enough that, in effect, all we had to do was steer. The trip was just great until the 24-mile mark when we hit a submerged branch, and in an instant the canoe had flipped and we were dumped into the water. The water was only mid-thigh, and after the initial shock we got ourselves back in the canoe and finished the trip.

Later when we were in the cabin, we both discovered that we had lost our wedding rings. Muriel was quite upset, but I convinced her that it was far more important that we were okay and we could always get new rings. When we returned the key to our hosts we were invited to stay overnight, and we got to sleep in their waterbed. After sleeping on a waterbed Muriel was hooked, and we eventually replaced our own bed with a waterbed. We shared that story back and forth, with me carrying the bulk of the telling, as we relived that wonderful time together. We did get new wedding bands, and we exchanged rings and renewed our vows on our 30th wedding anniversary.

Sunday, May 18, 2003

I went to church today only because Muriel said she would be okay while I was away. I was reluctant to leave her, but once again she insisted that it would be best for me to get away. So I waited until the last minute to depart and as soon as the service was over I returned home. She was fast asleep when I got back. I called both of our kids and shared with them that I think the end is near. They were both sad and asked me to keep them posted regarding their mother's condition.

Monday, May 19, 2003

Jackie was at our house early this morning, as I was scheduled to play golf with our regular foursome that played on Monday mornings. I had missed the first couple of these outings in the month and had gotten a substitute. However, last Wednesday I had told my friends I would be playing today. So I explained everything to Jackie, and since she had been here several times she pretty much knew the routine. I climbed the stairs and gave Muriel all of her medications for the morning, kissed her goodbye, and left her in Jackie's care. I was back by 2:00 and got a report from Jackie. Muriel had eaten her lunch but did not want to have a bath or her hair washed. Muriel had been talkative this morning and expressed an interest in how Jackie was doing in college and other aspects of her life. Jackie said she didn't make much sense at times, but she talked with her as best as she could.

After Jackie had left, I called Dr. Kretchmer's office. Muriel had an appointment scheduled for Tuesday and I canceled it.

When Muriel had finished dinner tonight she asked, "How are the kids?" Since I had called both of them on Sunday I had a ready report. I also said, "Neither Mark nor Kay will be present when you die."

"I think they should be here to comfort you."

"I'll be okay, and besides, it would be difficult for them to just come up here and stand by waiting for you to die. They don't live in the next town. They live a 2-day journey from us." She drifted off to sleep and that was the last time we discussed the matter.

Tuesday, May 20, 2003

We have reached the stage where Muriel is sleeping more, and I bide my time in the family room with my ear tuned to the receiver to be ready if she needs me. She is still eating, but each time it seems to be a little less. Barbara Christie, who was subbing for Susan, came by a little before 2:00 to check on Muriel. She took Muriel's vital signs as usual: pulse (92) and blood pressure (128/72).

When Barbara was finished Muriel was eager to tell her, "I weighed 113 pounds after my shower on Saturday."

It took some time for Muriel to say that and Barbara waited patiently for her to finish and then responded, "Well that's great. How are your pain levels?"

Muriel slurred out the words, "It seems like a two for both the ribs and the back as well as the liver area."

"How often are you using the Roxanol?"

I jumped in with, "It is most often at the end of the MS Contin cycle, and generally I gave her about 40 or maybe 60 cc. What we are concerned about right now is the lack of a bowel movement since Monday."

"You should try and increase the fluids she is taking, and today I want you to give her one Senocot. Starting tomorrow, give her the Senocot twice a day."

Thursday, May 22, 2003

I had gotten a substitute for my golf league yesterday and Muriel was upset with me and insisted that I play bridge today. Jackie came at 11:00 and I chatted with her until it was time for Muriel's lunch, and left that task for Jackie to assist her. I was back by 4:00 and Jackie reported that she had tried to provide companionship, but Muriel dozed off periodically.

In the evening she has the TV on continuously but oftentimes dozes off while it is on. After she has her midnight pill I always suggest she turn off the TV so I can get some sleep, since the sound is picked up by the monitoring system. I told her I need to get my rest to be ready to care for her. Generally she has been good about turning it off. At other times I just try to block it out as I want her to be free to watch something if she is awake. For some time she has had the light on all night, which is important if she wakes during the night and needs to use the commode next to the bed.

Sunday, May 25, 2003

I didn't go to church today, although Muriel wanted me to. I made the judgment that it was more important to be with her in the event she needed me. We had been concerned about Muriel not having a bowel movement when Barbara had been here on Tuesday, and the administration of the Senocot did the trick. It is no wonder that there is a problem, as she seems to be eating less and less. The pain seems to be more prevalent as the cycle of the MS Contin winds down, and she is taking more and more Roxanol. Way back, she had made me promise that she would be devoid of pain as her life ebbed away, and I have tried to be there to administer the liquid morphine when the stabbing pains arise.

She is sleeping more, but when she is awake we are able to carry on a conversation. Her responses are somewhat garbled at times and I have to try and figure out what she is trying to say. Thus, I tend to do most of the talking while she listens. I hold hands with her, help her to brush her teeth, wash her up and down, and then rub her with lotion. Because of the strenuous breathing involved it is almost impossible to have her get into the shower. She has not made any request for me to take her back to the hospice care center, so I judge I am doing a satisfactory job of caring for her.

Pastor Larry stopped by this afternoon to see Muriel, as well as me since I hadn't been in church in the morning. He did not stay very long and after reading scripture and saying prayers, he departed.

Wednesday, May 28, 2003

After I had given Muriel her medications this morning she gave me a jaundiced look. "I know you are upset with me this morning because I got a sub to play for me in my golf league." In addition, I have not been playing bridge on a regular basis. "I judge it is important that I be here to care for you." In her slurring pattern, she said, "Someone else, Lois or Jackie or Robin, can sit with me just as well."

"Muriel, my dear heart and love of my life, can you even imagine how I would feel if you died while I was playing golf or bridge? I would find it hard to forgive myself for not being here."

She was back with her usual argument. "We don't know when I am going to die and you need to get out."

"Okay, I'll call Lois to come Monday and I promise to go play golf."

After spending several days confined to her bed, at around 11:00 Muriel voiced her request on the monitor. "I want to come downstairs." I climbed the stairs and said, "I don't think that's a good idea. You know what a difficult time we'll have getting you back up here at the end of the day." But she insisted, so I upped her oxygen level to five liters per minute and got her into the wheelchair and brought her to the top of the stairs. She sat on the top step of the stairs while I folded the wheelchair and took it to the bottom to be ready to transport her to the family room. She moved her feet step by step as she slipped from one riser to the next on her backside. When she reached the bottom I helped her into the wheelchair and took her into the family room. Between the two of us she finally was seated in her recliner.

There was a sense of triumph on her part that if she was going to die, she was going to go out fighting and not just fold her tent. Once she was situated she wanted to see the movie *Love Among the Ruins* with Sir Laurence Olivier and Katharine Hepburn, a great "feel good" movie, and one of our favorites. I sat next to her in a matching recliner and we held hands as we watched the movie unfold. I don't know how much of the movie she actually saw but as the story developed I couldn't stop the tears from streaming down my cheeks.

Shortly after the movie ended, Suzanne Hamrick from VNS stopped by to administer to Muriel. I think she was surprised to see Muriel in the family room. A check of her vital signs indicated a slight elevation in the pulse (100), blood pressure at (132/62), and respirations at (26). Pain levels for all three areas were at the zero level at the time of the visit. We are getting low on a couple of medications so Suzanne called Dr. Koenig's office to have them fax an order to the pharmacy.

She listened to her breathing and suggested that Roxanol be used to help not only with Muriel's pain, but also with her breathing problems. She explained that the Roxanol would relax her and allow her to breathe more easily, helping to relieve her shortness of breath.

Oftentimes on Sunday mornings, especially during the cold winter months, when we had returned from church I would make us waffles, and tonight for dinner she wanted to have waffles which I lovingly prepared. I always preferred maple syrup, but Muriel had also stocked boysenberry, raspberry, and apple cinnamon. She chose boysenberry, so I fed her a nice warm waffle with boysenberry syrup and sips of coffee along the way.

After we had watched the news, I was ready to reverse the process of getting Muriel back upstairs. However, even before we began the process I gave her 40 cc of Roxanol in the interest of permitting easier breathing. I also turned the oxygen level up to five liters per minute. Then we began, out of the recliner and into the wheelchair, then I moved the wheelchair to the foot of the stairs. I helped her get out of the wheelchair and she leaned against the stair post while I moved the wheelchair to the top of the stairs. The first three or four steps were generally negotiated with little difficulty, but then the effort to breathe took over and the final six steps were negotiated one painful step at a time. Step, pause, gasp, gasp, repeat, until we finally made it to the top and back into the wheelchair. I have often volunteered to carry her up the stairs but she would not allow me to do that. I don't know if she thinks I might drop her or whether she thinks I might hurt myself if I tried. I wheeled Muriel next to the bed, but she just wanted to sit for a while before making the effort to get into bed. I think, all told, it was almost half an hour from the time we began the transporting process until Muriel was stretched out in bed. She dozed off almost immediately and I tiptoed downstairs.

I awakened her at 12:00 to administer her pills and she seemed to perk up briefly. I took a brief moment to pray with her and for her and to read the prayer "On Dying." She declared, "I love you," and I responded, "I love you too, so very, very much." The tears just streamed down my cheeks as we held hands in the silence of the moment. It gets more difficult each day as she continues to slip away.

Thursday, May 29, 2003

Muriel slept the night through and in the morning, I waited downstairs to hear her first stirrings. When she had not awakened by 8:00, I went upstairs to get her up for her morning pills. As I went up the stairs the thought was in the back of my mind that perhaps she had died overnight, but the minute I walked into the room I could tell she was breathing. I had brought a cup of coffee upstairs with me and I gently tried to rouse her. She seemed reluctant to awaken. Perhaps all of the effort of yesterday had taken its toll on her cancer-ridden body

•

and it wasn't a case of reluctance, she was just unable to awaken. I took the cup of coffee and returned downstairs. I didn't want to wait too long before she took her medications, but judged letting her continue to rest was better. She finally called for me at quarter to nine and I raced upstairs to minister to her needs. I helped her to use the commode at the bedside and then had her take her pills. "I want to brush my teeth."

"Okay sweetheart, let's brush teeth." So I got her toothbrush, a glass of water, and the spit trough we had salvaged from an earlier hospital visit. It was a slow process but successfully completed. I read to her from *Portals of Prayer* and thanked God for her and the life we share together, and then prayed for her to have a comfortable day. By then, she had dozed off again and I returned downstairs. I was having regrets that I let her come downstairs yesterday because I think the effort really taxed her system. However when the love of your life, who is dying, wants to make a trip downstairs you do all you can to make it happen.

Muriel was quiet most of the day. I had to awaken her at 4:00 to have her take the scheduled medications, and I also managed to get some food into her, part of a homemade muffin and a little fruit. I judge that because of their continuing work with cancer patients, the people at hospice are aware when a particular patient is close to death, because at close to 5:30 Cheryl Jansen, another nurse from VNS, stopped by to check on Muriel.

Muriel was pretty lethargic as Cheryl went about checking her vital signs. She reported, "Muriel's heart rate has increased and is at an irregular rate."

"She went downstairs yesterday and we had the Herculean task of getting her back up here because of the difficulty she had breathing. It probably took us almost a half hour to get her from her recliner to her bed."

"Did you give her any Roxanol?"

"We had not been doing that, but Suzanne mentioned it on her last visit and yesterday was the first time that I gave Muriel Roxanol to ease her breathing rather than for any breakthrough pain she might be experiencing."

"She is exhibiting signs of dying, but I can't say with any certainty that it is imminent. Do you want to have her return to the hospice care center where she will be regularly monitored?"

"No, Muriel seems comfortable under my care and I want her to be at home for now."

"I can have a hospital bed here tomorrow morning for her use."

"Thank you, but I think she is very comfortable in her waterbed. I'll think about all of these things over the weekend."

Friday, May 30, 2003

What a difference a day makes. Muriel was awake before 8:00 this morning and was ready for her pills when I arrived at her bedside. She greeted me with, "I'd like a cup of coffee." So I returned to the kitchen, happy to accommodate her request. I also made her a piece of toast, which she nibbled on until it was gone. I helped to get her propped up in bed and she seemed to be content to just watch television and doze off and on. I sat with her and held her hand. There was no talk of going downstairs, and even if she had requested it, I would not have permitted her to make the trip. After a lunch that consisted of a muffin and fruit she wanted to rest. A little before 3:00 Suzanne Hamrick stopped by to check up on her and I gently awakened her. Suzanne began to assess the vital statistics: pulse (80), blood pressure (118/72), and respirations (24). She listened to her heart and lungs and recorded that her breathing was labored. Current pain levels at the time of the visit were all recorded as zero. I think Suzanne was a little surprised at how alert Muriel was, as I am sure she had been informed of her state the prior two days. So there was nothing said about Muriel being close to death.

< 17 >
THE ADVENTURE COMES TO AN END

Sunday, June 1, 2003

Yesterday Muriel spent a quiet day, and nothing untoward happened. All of her medications were taken on time and there was no incidence of breakthrough pain. She slept much of the day. At dinnertime I brought her half of a muffin and some fruit. I propped her up so I could feed her. When that was accomplished, she slurred, "Do you plan on going to church in the morning?"

I was amazed that she knew it was Saturday and replied, "I feel I need to be here with you in case you need me."

She then asked, "Do you plan on playing golf on Monday?"

"Yes, I plan on playing golf on Monday. I have made arrangements to have Lois come and be with you while I am out." I tried to give her food, but she ate very little and was soon back to sleep.

Around 11:00 this morning Henrietta Wolf called to see if she could bring over a meal for us, and I assured her that we would welcome it. It wasn't the first time that people in our congregation have brought food. I recognized that it was their way of saying, "We care and we want to help you through this difficult time." The members of our church family have been unbelievably supportive through this whole adventure.

I spent time in the family room and when I heard Muriel stir upstairs I went up to hold her hand and stroke her face. I said, "I love you. I think you're hanging in there for me, but if you're ready to go and be with the Lord, it's okay with me." She just smiled back at me. The medications just make her so groggy, but she is apparently pain-free. The day just slipped by with no significant change. I went to bed with the thought that I should cancel Lois's visit tomorrow and not play golf. On the other hand, I had promised her that I would go play, and I want to honor that promise. In addition, Lois is an RN and will be able to handle any situation that might arise.

Monday, June 2, 2003

I was up a little after 7:00 and was eating breakfast when Lois arrived. Muriel awakened about quarter to eight and both Lois and I went up to greet her. I also brought up her medications which I had her take. I left her with Lois while I made preparations to leave for golf. When I went back to kiss her goodbye I could see residue of pills around her mouth and asked, "Have you swallowed all of your pills?"

She gave a barely audible, "Yes, I have."

"Please open your mouth." She complied and I could see further evidence that she had not completely swallowed all of her medications. "Please take another sip of water and swish it around in your mouth and then swallow." She seemed reluctant to do that, but she did take the sip of water and seemingly swished the remainder of the pills away. I kissed her goodbye and said, "Lois will be with you while I'm away." I told Lois, "I have my cell phone with me. If you need me, please call."

I drove to the golf course and played 18 holes, but I don't even remember what my score was for the day. I know it was not very good, as my mind was not really on swinging a golf club. When I finished my round I rushed home to relieve Lois and continue caring for Muriel. Lois said, "Muriel has eaten some fruit and had another cup of coffee, but mainly she slept."

"Thanks for staying and watching over her." She waved a goodbye, walked downstairs, and departed.

At 4:00 Muriel was due for another round of medications, especially the 300 mg of MS Contin which is primarily controlling the pain. When I went to give them to her she refused to take them. "Come on sweetheart, you need to take your medications." I tried the old childhood approach. "Pretty please, with sugar on it." All my coaxing was to no avail as she would not open her mouth. I then reminded her of the promise she had asked me to keep. "You wanted to be pain-free at the end of your life and you really need to take your pills."

She replied in barely a whisper, "I'm okay, I just don't want to take the pills." I finally decided that she knew what she was doing and I would just accept that. She wanted no dinner and she continued to sleep off and on. I called hospice and talked with Barbara Baird, and indicated that Muriel had essentially refused to take all of her medications. She suggested that I administer the medications through a suppository, but I was reluctant to do that so she said I should use the liquid morphine to relieve her pain. She suggested that I bring her to the hospice care center, but I told her it would be okay if Muriel dies at home. She said that she would have someone call me later.

I sat with her through the evening with the TV on in the background and the sound on mute. I got a warm washcloth and washed her face and hands and the upper part of her body. I talked to her about the good times we had shared together. "Do you remember the trip we took to England, where we visited all of the castles and Poets' Corner at Westminster Abbey?" Her eyes seemed to brighten as she thought about what I had said. *Does she remember? I have no idea.*

I reminded her about all of the Marriage Encounter weekends we had done as a team couple and how, together, we had affected the lives of other couples on the weekend. One of the talks we gave on the weekend when we were an administrative couple was about dying, and when Muriel gave her presentation there was not a dry eye in the place. "Do you recall giving your description of dying to those couples? You told them that it is like going away on a train but I am not going with you. You said that you could see me on the platform as the train pulled out of the station and there was no way you could pull me on board, and I just kept getting smaller and smaller until you couldn't see me anymore." I think she had some recollection because I could see tears run down her cheeks as I related the talk. I too was now crying uncontrollably. I gently wiped her tears away as we held hands and acknowledged the silent bond that exists between us. "I love you, Muriel." She seemed to mouth the words in return.

Hospice care called around 11:00 and I reported that all is well. They assured me that someone will stop by in the morning to check on Muriel. At midnight, she again refused to take her medications and I didn't even try to push it. I gave her a kiss goodnight and went to bed.

Tuesday, June 3, 2003

I was awakened at 2:00 when my monitor relayed the gut-wrenching cries of Muriel in great pain. I was instantly awake and rushed into the bedroom to see her writhing in pain on the bed and groaning and entreating me to help her get rid of the pain. "Keith, take the pain away." I felt so very helpless. Giving her pills at this time was out of the question, so I got 120 cc of liquid morphine and managed to get the dropper into her mouth and dispense the liquid. I refilled the dropper and repeated the process almost immediately. After about three or four minutes she began to calm down, and after ten minutes I had her ingest an additional 80 cc of the morphine. Throughout the ordeal she seemed to have some difficulty swallowing and that, perhaps, was the reason for not taking the pills earlier.

I stayed with her, seated in a chair next to the bed, in the event she needed me to administer additional doses of the liquid morphine. Periodically she would stir and groan, but it never seemed to be great enough to warrant an additional dosage. About 6:00 I went downstairs to have a cup of coffee and wash my face and hands. I ate a bowl of cereal and I also popped a muffin into the microwave and heated it up. I carried the muffin and the coffee upstairs to continue my vigil at her bedside. At 7:00 the groans and the writhing seemed to increase, so I gave her another 80 cc of the morphine. Suzanne Hamrick arrived at 8:20 and immediately gave Muriel 300 mg of MS Contin rectally and 200 mg of liquid morphine orally. She took her blood pressure (148/84), pulse (130), and respirations (28), listened to her heart and lungs, and told me that her heartbeat was irregular. Suzanne said, "Muriel is definitely exhibiting signs of dying, and I suggest that she be taken to the hospice care center where she can be monitored and properly medicated." At this stage I don't want to see Muriel suffer anymore and said, "I think that's a good idea." Suzanne took out her cell phone and called for an ambulance to transport Muriel to the hospice care center.

The ambulance arrived ten minutes later, without fanfare. There were three EMTs, two men and one woman. They brought a gurney to the front porch and the two men proceeded upstairs. I had come downstairs to let them in and remained at the bottom of the stairs waiting for them to bring Muriel down. I had anticipated that they would take the stretcher upstairs and return with Muriel on it, and was not prepared for what I saw next. They had rolled Muriel onto a sheet and then each of the medical technicians rolled up two corners, and down the stairs they came with Muriel slung between them. All I could think of was a picture of an earlier culture bringing home a carcass slung on a pole between two men. It is an image that will stick with me, and not a very pleasant one. My wife was leaving our home for the last time like a sack of potatoes. Admittedly, they were very gentle with her and placed her lovingly on the gurney. They quickly covered her with blankets, strapped her to the gurney, placed her in the ambulance, and departed for the hospice care center out in Fairlawn. Suzanne had followed the technicians down the stairs and indicated that she had called the center. They would be expecting Muriel's arrival and had a room waiting for her. Suzanne expressed her condolences and departed. There I stood in the middle of the living room with tears streaming down my cheeks. Muriel will never be back in this house ever again. It is extremely difficult to contemplate. I pulled myself together, took a quick shower, dressed, got some reading material, and drove to the hospice care center.

I checked at the nurse's station to determine in which room Muriel had been placed. The room is very similar to the one that Muriel had occupied when she was there in April. The curtains in the room had been drawn and the only light present is a fluorescent panel light behind the bed. Muriel lay in the bed hooked up to the oxygen with her arms outside the covers and looks so very peaceful. I didn't know whether additional medications had been given when she arrived or whether the medications that Suzanne had administered were the ones controlling her pain. Ten minutes later a nurse walked in the room and asked, "What is your name?" I said, "I am Keith Klafehn, husband of Muriel Klafehn who is lying here in this bed."

"Are there any other members of the family coming?"

"No, it will just be me."

Her next words sent a chill up my spine. "Muriel is dying. Signs were observed when she was brought in. She has been given an additional intravenous shot of morphine after she was settled in her bed."

I said, "Thank you for the information," and watched her walk out the door.

I stood next to Muriel's bed, leaning over the railing, and stroked her face. Once again I said, "I love you sweetheart. It's okay if you want to go to be with the Lord, but if you want to stay, I will be happy to spend more time with you." I wanted to think she smiled at me but I don't even know if she heard me. I took a break from just being with her and called the church. "Hello, this is Redeemer. May I help you?"

I recognized the secretary's voice and said, "Rita, it's Keith. I am calling to let you know that Muriel was taken to the hospice care center this morning, and it is pretty certain she won't be coming back home."

"Oh Keith, I am so sorry for you."

"Thanks, Rita. Please let Pastor Johnson and Pastor Larry know."

"I certainly will. Thank you for calling and letting us know."

At noontime Pastor Johnson and Ann Bolf arrived. Ann had been in the office when I had called Rita and decided immediately that she wanted to come out to lend support. I got a big hug from Ann and a handshake from Pastor Johnson. We talked briefly about Muriel's prognosis and the fact that she is dying. We assembled around the bed and Pastor Johnson said prayers of thanksgiving for Muriel's life and her dedication to all of the Lord's work in our church, and to her faith, which had been a gift to many of the people in the congregation. He prayed that her pain be diminished and that she have a peaceful release from this life, and arrive safely in the mansions in Heaven. Muriel's peace that she had prayed for at the outset of this adventure just permeated the room and enveloped us all.

After Pastor Johnson and Ann departed, I stopped at the nurse's station and determined that Muriel's death is not imminent, so I informed her that I was going home for a brief time but would come right back. The one-way trip is about 12 miles, and when I got home I called both of our children to let them know their mom was at the hospice care center. I was able to talk to Mark and I left a message for Kay. I also called Muriel's sister Judith and passed on the same information. I made myself a peanut butter sandwich, grabbed the memorial service folder that Muriel had prepared, and immediately headed back to the center.

I arrived back midafternoon and Muriel was just as I had left her. I spent the rest of the afternoon just holding her hand and being there as her life ebbed away. At 6:00 I left her briefly to have a bowl of the chicken noodle soup that the Lutheran ladies had supplied the care center and ate in silence in the kitchen. When I finished I poured myself a cup of coffee and returned to the room to maintain my vigil.

During the afternoon a nurse had given Muriel another shot of morphine, and at 8:00 another nurse—there had been a shift change—came to administer medications orally with a dropper. I was not quick enough to stop her and for a moment it looked like Muriel was going to choke on the liquid. The nurse immediately realized the problem and began to syringe the liquid away. When Muriel was all calmed down she proceeded to provide the morphine intravenously. Around 10:00 I began to sing to Muriel. I sang hymns. I sang pop tunes. I sang nursery rhymes. I sang songs from many of the musical shows we are familiar with. I sang the songs that we had grown up with during our courtship. Sometimes there was just a *la la la* as the words did not come back to me.

Wednesday, June 4, 2003

I continued my singing into a new day but my voice was beginning to weaken. I took a break and began to look through the memorial service folder and discovered that all four of the poems that she wanted read at her memorial service were in the folder. Since, obviously, they were four of her favorites, I decided to read each of them to her. I began with "Advice to My Son" by J. Peter Meinke. This was followed by the *Holy Sonnets* by John Donne. Next came Shakespeare's *Cymbeline*, Act 4, Scene 2, starting with line 258. The last reading was entitled "Fern Hill." It is a poem by Dylan Thomas, one of her all-time favorite authors. When I finished reading the last poem, Muriel took a deep breath, exhaled, and the adventure had come to an end.

I thought she had died, so I left the room and went to the nurse's station. The nurse on duty greeted me with, "Can I help you?"

"Yes, I think my wife has just died."

The nurse left the desk immediately and I followed her back to Muriel's room, where she confirmed that indeed Muriel had died. The nurse gave me a big hug and said, "You can stay with her as long as you want." Before she departed she asked, "Who is to do the funeral arrangements?" I gave her the information and then went back to the bedside and gazed at her lifeless body. She looked so different. I gently picked up each of her hands and placed them under the covers. I thought of the three songs that we had treasured during our courtship and beyond. The first line of "The Twelfth of Never" immediately came to mind: "You ask how much I need you, must I explain? I need you, oh my darling, like roses need rain." Through the years we so enjoyed each other's company and now it was "Softly as I Leave You." I cradled her head in my hands and kissed her on the forehead and then walked silently to the parking lot.

I had a CD in my car of the solo piano works of Danny Wright, and as I drove home I alternated between two tracks, "Softly as I Leave You" by Henry Mancini and "Where is Love?" from *Oliver*. As I drove I couldn't stop the tears from flowing. When I got home I went right to bed. All of the necessities associated with a death can wait until the morning.

I wrote a poem for Muriel on the occasion of her 50th birthday and it seems appropriate at the close of her life.

Upon Becoming Fifty

There is standard time
And light saving time,
And digits and dials that tell us time;
There's a magazine Time
And stitches in time,
And when we do nothing we call it mark time;
There is high time
And noontime,
And tummies that tell us that now it's mealtime;
We stretch time
And squeeze time,
And then there are days we run out of time;
On our hands we have time
And now is the time,
And we leave the door open when we say anytime;
We have daytime
And nighttime,
And the end of the day brings us bedtime;
We post time
And steal time,
And between now and then, there is meantime;
There's a right time
And a wrong time,
And when imprecise, we label it sometime;
There is pastime
And real time,
And events in our life are moments in time;
But should moments be lost
And pass from out view,
Or should we recall
How time fazes you;
You take time to listen
And you give time to care;
Whether friends or with family, you have time to share
And I love you.
You take time for music
And you seek time to read;

Whether learning or pleasure, it is time that you need
And I love you.
You take time for planning
And you give time to cook;
Whether fish, chicken, turkey, you spend time to look
And I love you.
You take time for walking
And you seek time to rest;
Whether morning or evening, it's time to look best
And I love you.
You've times when you're up
And times when you're low
Whether topside or bottom, it's a time that you grow
And I love you.
You take time for earning
And you make time to spend;
Whether bargains or needs, it's the time that you blend
And I love you.
You find time to laugh
And hide time to cry;
Whether snickers or sniffles, it's a time to pass by
And I love you.
You take time to worship
And you seek time for fun;
Whether movies or golfing, or time in the sun
And I love you.
You like time for loving
And you like time to be;
But all times together are the best times for me.
And I love you.

< 18 >
EPILOGUE

Monday, June 9, 2003

THE CELEBRATION OF THE LIFE, DEATH,
AND RESURRECTION OF
MURIEL E. J. KLAFEHN
CHILD OF GOD, WIFE, MOTHER, GRANDMOTHER, FRIEND

That is the way the bulletin read that was passed out at Muriel's memorial service. Both of our children with their families, my two sisters from Florida, numerous friends from church, from Muriel's support group, from her university associations, and neighbors were in attendance. The service was exactly as she had designed it from start to finish. She would have been pleased. There was just one change. Lois Jenkins had been designated to read one of the poems but had to work, so Kay's husband, Larry, became the reader.

Muriel had chosen several scripture passages to be read and it seems fitting that one of them was the passage from Isaiah 40:31, *"But those who hope in the Lord will renew their strength. They will soar on wings like eagles; they will run and not grow weary, they will walk and not be faint."* She had begun her adventure soaring on wings of eagles and she ends her adventure in the same manner.

The final scripture reading she had selected comes from 2nd Timothy 4:7, "I have fought the good fight, I have finished the race, I have kept the faith." Throughout her adventure she was a rock and never wavered in the belief that God had permitted her to have cancer so she could be a living message to all she met, that believing in the Lord Jesus Christ will sustain you.

As a congregation, we sang "Love Divine, All Love Excelling," a hymn that had been sung at our wedding as well as the wedding of our daughter. The Chorale, that she had so faithfully directed, sang all three selections that she had chosen.

Pastor Larry delivered a eulogy which ended with "most I will remember Muriel as a dear friend, a compassionate caregiver, and an indomitable spirit." Pastor Johnson delivered the sermon based on a text that Muriel had chosen. It is from St. Paul's Letter to the Romans, 8:38-39, "For I am convinced that neither death nor life, neither angels nor demons, neither the present nor the future, nor any powers, neither height nor depth, nor anything else in all creation, will be able to separate us from the love of God that is in Christ Jesus our Lord."

Towards the end of Pastor Johnson's sermon he said, "Muriel went to Heaven while her husband Keith was singing to her. He mentioned to us one of the verses from 'The Servant Song:' 'I will hold the Christ light for you / In the night time of your fear / I will hold my hand out to you / Speak the peace you long to hear.' That word of peace has been pronounced upon Muriel. She is now home in Heaven. Jesus Christ won her for Himself. He claimed her for Himself. And He has now received her home to Himself. There is nothing now that will ever be able to separate Muriel from the love of God, which is in Christ Jesus the Lord. Amen!"

It seemed so fitting that the peace which Muriel had prayed for at the beginning of her adventure was now pronounced upon her as a climax to her life.

We celebrated Holy Communion and the recessional hymn was entitled "Shine, Jesus, Shine." Muriel had selected it especially for me as she knew it was one of my all-time favorites. I always cry when I sing it and today it was a total wipeout considering the context of the hymn.

There was a dinner after the service and I think nearly all of the persons who attended the service came by to pay homage to Muriel and to offer comfort to me and our family. One of the last things I did before going in to eat was to present Sue d'Amico, who had taken care of all of the music and directed the Chorale for the service, with the soaring eagle pin that I had given to Muriel near the beginning of her adventure. She wanted Sue to have it.

Thursday, August 7, 2003

Today I honored Muriel's final request. Kay, our daughter, and Kenton, our grandson, were also in attendance when Pastor Gnewuch of Risen Christ Lutheran Church in North Myrtle Beach conducted a private service on the beach, with the waves lapping at our feet, to inter Muriel's mortal remains. We did this by spreading her ashes in the waters of the Atlantic Ocean. And Muriel's final wish was fulfilled!

Friday, May 20, 2005

Today, Frances I. Krzak of Belle Vernon, Pennsylvania and I were married by Pastor Larry in the privacy of his office. It was a fulfillment of Muriel's admonition to me in the last days of her life "to get on with your life, go find someone new and get married." Frances had lost her husband in 1996, so we were two individuals who had lost a spouse and found each other.

Muriel's adventure encompassed four years, eight months, and twelve days. The total expense that was chargeable during this time frame was $245,355.19. In the table shown below I have provided all the pertinent statistics related to Muriel's care.

CATEGORY	TOTAL
Number of doctors associated with her care	38
Number of doctor's appointments	97
Number of times blood pressure taken	102
Number of needle sticks	68
Number of times her pulse was taken	60
Number of times she was weighed	57
Number of radiation treatments	68
Number of respiration recordings	42
Number of blood tests taken	36
Number of medications prescribed	38
Number of visitations by personnel from VNS	37
Number of IVs	29

CATEGORY	TOTAL
Number of times temperature was taken	17
Number of Aredia treatments	19
Number of chemotherapy sessions	8
Number of CT scans	7
Number of bone scans	6
Number of MUGA scans	2
Number of days in the hospital	8
Number of days at the hospice care center	11
Number of chest X-rays	10
Number of mammograms	3
Number of gynecological visits	3
Number of visits by home health care aides	7
Number of oxygen saturation tests recorded	5
Number of mastectomies	2
Number of colonoscopies	2
Number of EKGs	1
Number of small bowel tests	1
Number of MRIs	1
Number of breathing tests	1
Number of port insertions	1
Number of port removals	1
Number of trips to the emergency room	1
Number of ambulance transports	1
Number of miles driven for all care	3824

ACKNOWLEDGMENTS

In the course of a prolonged illness there are many individuals who assist in the care of the person involved. I wish to pay tribute to all the doctors who were intimately involved with Muriel's care during this time, especially Dr. James Waugh, Dr. Daniel Abood, and Dr. Michael Maggio, her primary care physicians; Dr. Joseph Koenig, her oncologist, who cared for her for nearly five years; Dr. John Karlen, gynecological oncologist; Dr. Michael Flynn, surgeon; Dr. Michael Cline, gastroenterologist; Dr. Desiree Doncals, radiation oncologist; Dr. Kenneth Kretchmer, pulmonologist; and Dr. Merideth Driscoll, physician at the hospice care center.

Additional thanks to the numerous doctors who read X-rays, CT scans, body scans, MUGA scans, and MRIs. Thank you to all of the technicians, whose expertise in the use of the equipment, provided all of the scans. The staff at Summit Oncology Associates were all so helpful, friendly, and extremely efficient in the tasks they performed, especially Beth Stein who never failed to find a vein with minimal duress to Muriel. Thank you to the staff at the hospice care center as well as the Visiting Nurse Service staff who attended Muriel at home, especially Susan Slagle, her regular nurse.

I want to thank all the members of Muriel's support group who were always there for her, especially Robin Graham, Sue Wells, and Linda Allen. I can't name all of the people in our congregation, but the support provided to both Muriel and me was overwhelming and for that I thank you. Donna Thrush and Betty Dodd get a special thank you for the card ministry throughout Muriel's "adventure." The visits by Pastor Larry, Pastor Al, and Pastor Johnson were greatly appreciated by both Muriel and me.

Thank you to Lois Jenkins and Sue Wells, who read early chapters of this book, and Christine Stroub and Michaelann Hammonds, who read the complete manuscript, for your suggestions.

Thanks to the publisher of the card "Anniversary Thoughts of the Day Our Love Began" by Michele Savicki, © 1993 by Blue Mountain Arts, Inc. All rights reserved. Reprinted with permission. Thanks also to American Greetings Corporation for permission to publish words from the birthday card we shared. Reproduced with permission. American Greetings Corporation © AGC, LLC.

Thanks to Music Services, Inc. for permission to publish an excerpt from Richard Gillard's "The Servant Song," © 1977 Scripture in Song/ Maranatha! Music/ASCAP. All rights administered by Music Services, Inc. All rights reserved. Used by permission. Thank you also to Lifetouch Church Directories and Portraits for permission to use the portrait of Muriel and me which appears on the cover of this book.

Thanks to Katii O'Brien and Roger Calado for their efforts in editing, proofreading, and preparing this book for publication. Lastly, a special thank you to Kate Lautens and Steve Furr, my author support representatives at Trafford Publishing, who held my hand and walked me through the publishing process to enable me to tell others of the journey that one person traveled on this "adventure" called cancer.

Printed in the United States
By Bookmasters